LOVE
IS THE
CURE

Sir Elton John is a renowned musician, songwriter, performer, and humanitarian. His five-decade career has included many achievements as a recording artist, as well as in theatre and film.

www.ejaf.org (US)
www.ejaf.com (UK)

Sales of LOVE IS THE CURE
benefit the Elton John AIDS Foundation.

LOVE
IS THE
CURE

ELTON JOHN

ON LIFE, LOSS, AND THE END OF AIDS

HODDER

First published in Great Britain in 2012 by Hodder & Stoughton
An Hachette UK company

First published in paperback in 2013

1

A CIP catalogue record for this title is available from the British Library

ISBN 978 1 444 75703 3

Typeset by Palimpsest Book Production Limited, Falkirk, Stirlingshire

Printed and bound by Clays Ltd, St Ives plc

Hodder & Stoughton policy is to use papers that
are natural, renewable and recyclable products and made from
wood grown in sustainable forests. The logging and manufacturing
processes are expected to conform to the environmental
regulations of the country of origin.

Hodder & Stoughton Ltd
338 Euston Road
London NW1 3BH

www.hodder.co.uk

In memory of Robert Key, a dear friend and tireless advocate for those living with HIV/AIDS around the world

CONTENTS

Foreword

Thirty years after the advent of the AIDS epidemic, what have we learned about this disease and about ourselves as human beings?

On the first score, there's cause for optimism about the power of scientific advancements and the potential for a new view of global health and clinical medicine. Three decades after the first cases of AIDS were reported, we have identified the virus that causes the syndrome and can block its replication. We have developed, and continue to improve, tools to diagnose and treat the disease. Astoundingly, we have delivered on some of these advances to millions of the poorest and sickest people in the world – in Africa, in Haiti, in the remotest corners of Asia.

But anyone wondering why, despite these advancements, there are still so many people living with HIV/AIDS today should read the book you now hold. Even for those familiar with the history of the epidemic, Elton

John's work is a revelation. Written by a man who helped form the soundtrack and spirit of a generation, Elton's book gives us a vision for the future that is both cautionary and inspiring.

Love is the Cure reflects just how deeply, and for how long, Elton has been committed to eradicating AIDS in settings as diverse the rural South in the United States, Haiti (where Elton's foundation has supported the work of Partners In Health), South Africa, and Ukraine. These are the front lines of the AIDS crisis today, and from the work in these settings around the world, we begin to see solutions emerge.

The story recounted in these pages is about this work and how a world-famous musician came to master its complexities. *Love is the Cure* is an honest account, grateful and graceful, told largely through the eyes of activists, caregivers, and AIDS patients who have struggled against this disease because they live on the margins of our society. What Elton has discovered through his commitment to ending AIDS is, perhaps, the closest thing we have to a panacea for poverty, preventable disease, and the despair we find in frightening abundance around the world: compassion that translates into action.

I'm writing this foreword at our office in Rwanda. At the close of 1994, following the genocide that took up to a million lives, Rwanda was in ruins. Many of its hospitals and clinics had been thoroughly damaged or destroyed; others were simply abandoned; a large portion of the health work force had been killed or languished in refugee camps. These settlements, especially those within Rwanda, were ravaged and thinned by cholera and other 'camp epidemics,' as well as by AIDS, tuberculosis, and malaria. Child mortality rates soared to the highest in the world; malnutrition was rampant. Many development experts were ready to write off this beleaguered nation as a lost cause, a failed state.

Today, two decades later, Rwanda is the only country in sub-Saharan Africa on track to meet, by 2015, each of the health-related development goals that almost all the world's countries agreed upon 13 years ago. More than 93 per cent of Rwandan infants are inoculated against eleven vaccine-preventable illnesses. Over the past decade, death during childbirth has declined by more than 60 per cent. Deaths attributed to AIDS, tuberculosis, and malaria have dropped even more steeply, as have all deaths registered among children under five. Rwanda is one of only two countries on the continent to achieve the goal of universal access to AIDS therapy; the other is far wealthier Botswana. There's still a long way to go. But these are some of the steepest declines in mortality ever documented, anywhere and at any time in recorded history.

If that's not a big-time reversal of fortune, I don't know what is.

This has come to pass for many reasons and with the help of many partners. Some of the improvement in Rwanda has occurred because the *global* pandemic of neglect is also being addressed. The U.S. government is far and away the largest single funder of AIDS treatment programs in Africa. Indeed, simply by doing the math we see that many Americans now support efforts to build programs that can save lives, improve health, and prevent discrimination in all its forms.

But Rwanda's rebirth has come to pass most of all because of good leadership here and sound policies in development, in public health, and in clinical medicine. It has come to pass because some of Rwanda's leaders, including its health minister, have joined civil society groups to fight discrimination with legal remedies, with activism, and with an effort to realise the right to care. And much of this improvement has occurred among the poor and in the country's rural reaches, traditionally neglected by governments and by medical professionals, but also by human rights groups and non-governmental organisations.

Building a proper health system offers care providers

the chance to be more effective and humane. Working as a doctor in places as far-ranging as a Harvard teaching hospital, a clinic in rural Haiti, and even a prison in Siberia has taught me something that Elton John learned by acting on his empathy, year after year and in country after country. Context matters and people are different, but they are much more the same. The aspirations of our patients – to receive care, to feel better, to be heard, to help friends and family members, to get back to work or to return to school – are universal. Too many of these aspirations are dashed not only by serious illness but also by local poverty and social inequalities of all sorts. All of these pathologies need to be attacked with resolve, resources, and a clear commitment to a human rights agenda that links our quest for a right to health care to respect for the rights of everyone to live free of any sort of persecution or disdain. This is how to battle stigma, as Elton documents so well in this book.

Love is the Cure is a crash course on the complexities of these mortal dramas. Some readers will be most interested in Elton's own quest for sobriety and a life of meaning; still others will want to know how all of this led to the creation of the Elton John AIDS Foundation, and how EJAF works. Most striking to me is the way Elton offers us a social history of the AIDS epidemic, which was, in more technical terms, a global pandemic, moving forward most quickly wherever poverty and social inequality and abuse of human rights form a noxious synergy. That's why pragmatic solidarity and the unstable sentiments that can inform it – from compassion to love – are so important to the future of our efforts to fight AIDS. It's why all of us can and should be involved. All of us, regardless of background, will one day need effective care just as we need respect and compassion. We cannot assume that others, including the AIDS activists to whom we owe a great deal, will do this hard work for us.

As Elton reminds us throughout this book, we cannot also assume that compassion and respect alone will yield a cure, let alone eradication of AIDS. Clear policies must be implemented on a global scale – policies that are effective, that save lives, and that can be scaled. We should all be haunted by the realisation that in many instances, the global community has decided, simply, not to fight this disease with the best weapons available. Elton John sounds a clarion call for compassion and empathy, but also for specific policies and actions that, without a doubt, will help us realise an AIDS-free generation, and perhaps eventually, an AIDS-free world.

Twenty years ago, Rwanda was the most troubled nation on Earth. Today, it is one of the most hopeful.

The work of Partners In Health, other activist groups, and all those striving to end AIDS has taught me that there is no such thing as a hopeless situation, no such thing as a lost cause. Such is the case with the AIDS epidemic at large. Elton understands intuitively, and personally, that with the hard work of advocates and experts, with the commitment of resources and political pressure, and above all, with compassion as our guiding principle, we can bring about an end to AIDS.

Love is the Cure is an essential polemic about how we reach the end of AIDS and eradicate this affliction. This can't happen in enduring ways without linking empathy or other transient emotions to pragmatic solidarity and social change, which, as Elton John makes so clear, is always informed by deep knowledge and discernment.

Paul Farmer, MD, PhD, Harvard University, Partners In Health
Kigali, Rwanda
June 24, 2013

I

Ryan

I've thought about this book for a while now, though it never occurred to me how to start off.

I suppose one could begin with statistics, with numbers and charts and facts that paint the perfect picture of horror that is the global AIDS epidemic: more than 25 million lives lost in thirty years, 34 million people living with HIV/AIDS around the globe, 1.8 million deaths per year, nearly 5,000 lives taken each and every day, the sixth leading cause of death worldwide.

But I've always found it impossible to comprehend these statistics. The tragedy is so immense, the figures are so enormous, there's simply no way to wrap your mind around it all.

Let's leave the numbers for later, and begin with a story instead.

After all, I'm not a statistician; I'm a musician. I've made my living telling stories through songs. It gives me incredible joy the way people connect with my music. That is all I hope to do in this book – to tell stories that connect people with this epidemic, so we can work together to end it.

The first story I'd like to tell you is an amazing one. To understand the AIDS epidemic, to understand my passion for ending it, you need to know about Ryan White. It all goes back to my friend Ryan.

Ryan came into this world with a rare and terrible genetic disease, haemophilia, which prevents the blood from clotting and leads to uncontrollable bleeding. Haemophilia is a manageable condition today, but in the early 1970s, when Ryan was born, it was a dangerous and often fatal disease. As an infant, and then as a child, Ryan was in the hospital again and again.

Then, as if the hand he'd been dealt wasn't difficult enough, the poor boy contracted HIV, the virus that causes AIDS, through a treatment for his haemophilia. At age thirteen, the doctors gave Ryan a grim prognosis: less than six months to live. He held on for more than five years. And in that short span, Ryan accomplished what most could not hope to achieve in a thousand lifetimes. He inspired a nation, changed the course of a deadly epidemic, and helped save millions of lives. Imagine, a child doing all of that, a sick boy from a small town in Middle America. It sounds like a movie script, like a bedtime story, like a miracle. And it was a miracle. Ryan's life was an absolute miracle.

It must have been 1985 when I first learned about Ryan. I was at a doctor's appointment in New York. I forget why I was there. I picked up a magazine from a stack in the waiting room. I was mindlessly flipping through the pages when I came across an article that would change my life. I couldn't believe what I was reading, that a boy was being kept out of school, and his family was being shunned and tormented, because he had AIDS.

Ryan lived with his mother, Jeanne, and his younger sister, Andrea, in the small town of Kokomo, Indiana. Jeanne worked at the local General Motors car factory for twenty-three years. The Whites were a blue-collar family through and through, much like my own family growing up, which is perhaps why I instantly connected with them when we finally got to know one another.

In 1984, around Christmastime, Ryan was in particularly bad shape with a rare form of pneumonia. But tests at the hospital revealed a far worse diagnosis: he had full-blown AIDS. The pneumonia was an opportunistic infection attacking his badly weakened immune system.

As it turned out, Ryan had contracted HIV from a

treatment for his haemophilia called factor VIII, a clotting agent derived from donated blood. A single dose of factor VIII could include plasma pooled from thousands of people, and some of them had HIV. Because the HIV virus itself wasn't identified until the mid-1980s, there was no way to screen for the disease. That's how HIV-contaminated factor VIII was administered to patients in the United States and throughout the world in the early '80s, including Ryan. Thousands of haemophiliacs became HIV-positive in this way before pharmaceutical companies and the government put measures in place to test and purify factor VIII.

Jeanne waited until after Christmas to tell Ryan that he had AIDS. When he found out, Ryan knew exactly what it meant: he was going to die.

Everyone was aware of AIDS by 1984, especially haemophiliacs. While it was still a very new and frightening disease, the medical community had already figured out the basics. They had identified the HIV virus itself that year, and they knew that it was spread only by sex or by direct blood exposure. More to the point, they knew it couldn't be transmitted through casual contact, such as sharing water fountains or toilet seats, drinking from the same glass, eating with the same utensils, or even kissing. There was simply no risk of infection from being around someone with AIDS.

4

But there was fear. There was so much fear. It was everywhere, a ghost that shadowed Ryan's every move and haunted him throughout his life.

When Ryan was told about his condition, that he might not have very long to live, he made an extraordinary decision: to live out the rest of his days, however many there might be, as ordinarily as he could. He wanted to go to school, to play with his friends, and to spend time with his mom, Andrea, and his grandparents. He just wanted to be like any other child, even if his disease meant that he wasn't. When he first learned of his prognosis, Ryan asked Jeanne to pretend that he didn't have AIDS. He didn't want special treatment; all he wanted was a sense, however brief, of normality.

But that would not be his fate. Ryan was never allowed to live a normal life, let alone die a normal death. Shortly after he was diagnosed, a local paper discovered that Ryan had AIDS. They ran a story about it, and suddenly the whole town – and then the whole nation – knew about his condition. After that, everything changed for Ryan and his family. As a child with haemophilia, Ryan had been treated with compassion. As a child with AIDS, many treated him with contempt.

Ryan missed the majority of seventh grade, thanks to his bout with pneumonia. He was too weak to return to school that year, in the spring of 1985. By the summer, however, he was much better. He even had a paper round. He was eager to be back in school, to play with his friends, to have a semblance of a normal life. But in late July, a month before the beginning of the new school year, the superintendent of Ryan's school district announced that Ryan would not be allowed to attend classes in person, due to the widespread fear that he posed a health risk to his schoolmates – that by being near them, he might somehow infect them. It was decided that Ryan would attend school by phone instead.

The fear, I suppose, was understandable. AIDS was a fatal illness at the time, without exception. But it was well known that Ryan couldn't transmit the virus to others just by being around them. After all, Jeanne and Andrea lived with Ryan. They drank out of the same glasses, ate off the same dishes, hugged him, kissed him. They were with him constantly, especially when he was most sick. Yet even their intimate proximity to Ryan hadn't resulted in their contracting HIV. Besides, the U.S. Centers for Disease Control and Prevention (CDC) and the Indiana State Board of Health had assured the school district that Ryan posed no threat to teachers, students, or staff, and they offered guidelines for him to safely return.

Logic and science couldn't contain the fear, however.

Ryan was effectively quarantined. But he wasn't a quitter; he never, ever gave up. Not being allowed to attend school was unacceptable to him. He decided to fight to return.

Ryan and Jeanne sued the school. They had the national medical community and the State Board of Health on their side. But the judge dismissed Ryan's lawsuit. He said that the boy's lawyers had to appeal the school superintendent's decision to the Indiana Department of Education first. Ryan's days were numbered as it was, and here was a technical decision that would further delay his going back to school. In the meantime, a special phone link was set up, and Ryan dialled into school every day.

The appeals process that ensued was long, nasty, and public, with Ryan, now fourteen years old, at the centre of it all. The local school board and many parents of Ryan's schoolmates were vehemently opposed to him attending school. More than a hundred parents threatened to file a lawsuit if Ryan was allowed to return. In late November, the Indiana Department of Education ruled in Ryan's favour and ordered the school to open its doors to him, except when he was very sick. The local school board appealed, prolonging Ryan's absence from the classroom. Months later, a state board again ruled that Ryan should be allowed to attend school with the approval of a county health official.

With more than half the school year gone, Ryan was officially cleared to return to classes on 21 February, 1986. The thrill of victory, though, was short-lived. On his first day back, he was pulled from the classroom and brought to court. A group of parents had filed an injunction to block his return, and the judge issued a restraining order against him. When the judge handed down his verdict, the room packed with parents began to cheer, while Ryan and Jeanne looked on, shocked and scared. It seemed like a modern-day witch hunt, and Ryan was to be burned at the stake.

Ryan's lawyers fought the restraining order, and he *again* won the right to go back to school. This time the decision was final. On 10 April, 1986, with hordes of press on his heels and some students picketing nearby, Ryan returned to classes. He was not allowed to participate in gym class, and he was made to use a separate bathroom and water fountain, and disposable utensils in the cafeteria. These were needless precautions, but Ryan agreed to them in order to assuage the fears about his misunderstood disease. Still, twenty-seven children were withdrawn from school that day. Two weeks later, parents opened an alternative school, and twenty-one of Ryan's schoolmates were enrolled so as not to be in the same building as Ryan daily.

Back at school, and nearly everywhere he went in his hometown, Ryan was teased and tormented. He was called a 'fag' and other homophobic obscenities in public. His school locker and possessions were vandalised, and terrible rumours were spread about him. One anonymous teenager wrote a letter to the local paper accusing Ryan of threatening to bite and scratch other children, spitting on food at a grocery store, even urinating on bathroom walls. These were lies, of course, but it didn't matter. Having AIDS made Ryan a freak, and regardless of what he did or didn't do, he was considered as such.

If you can believe it, adults treated him even worse than children did. People on Ryan's paper round cancelled their subscriptions. When he and his family went out to eat, local restaurants would throw away the dishes they used. The parents of Ryan's girlfriend forbade her from seeing him. At one point during the Whites' legal battle with the school district, a group of school parents demanded that the county declare Jeanne an unfit guardian in order to have Ryan taken away from her, and thus taken out of school.

It wasn't just Ryan who was subjected to ill treatment and ostracism – his entire family suffered. The tyres were slashed on Jeanne's car. A bullet was shot through a window of the White family's home. Ryan's extended family was harassed, too, and even non-relatives who defended Ryan were subjected to abuse. When the local paper supported Ryan's right to attend school, the publisher's house was egged. A reporter at the paper even received death threats.

Somehow, Ryan's disease brought out the very worst in people, and there was little refuge for him and his family. Not even at church. The Whites were people of deep faith and Christian convicition. Each night, Ryan and Jeanne prayed together before bed. But after Ryan's illness became public, the community at their Methodist church began to shun them. The parishioners were so afraid of catching AIDS from Ryan that he and his family were asked to sit in either the first pew or the last. People wouldn't use the church bathroom after Ryan. Parents told their children to avoid him.

In his autobiography, Ryan tells the story of his family going to church on Easter Sunday in 1985, shortly after his diagnosis. At the end of the service, people turned to those sitting around them to shake hands and say, 'Peace be with you,' an Easter tradition at Ryan's church. No one would shake his hand this time. Not a single person would offer this sick child a blessing of peace on Easter. As they left the church that morning, Jeanne's car broke down. She tried to stop members of the congregation leaving the church car park, but no one would help her.[1]

Despite the ostracism he suffered from his church and his community, and despite the terrible pain and physical distress he experienced his entire life, Ryan was full of faith and Christian love until the end. Only a year before he died, Ryan told the *Saturday Evening Post* that he wasn't afraid of dying because of his faith in God. Even after he had endured so much abuse from fraudulent zealots, and as he was growing sicker, Ryan's faith was stronger than ever. 'There's always hope with the Lord,' Ryan told the *Post*. 'I have a lot of trust in God.'[2]

As a boy, I loved Sunday school. I loved hearing stories from the Bible, stories full of hope. To this day, while I do not practise any religion, I do take the compassionate teachings of Jesus to heart, and I have great respect for all people of faith. I am inspired by Jesus the man because he loved unconditionally, because he forgave unconditionally, and because he died for the sake of others. The same can be said of Ryan White. He was a true Christian, a modern-day Jesus Christ. That's a bold statement, I know; some might even take offence to it. But to know Ryan's story, and to have witnessed his extraordinary qualities as I did, is to come to no other conclusion.

The White family put their Christian faith to practice. They were upset at being treated so terribly by their community, of course, but they understood the fear. They knew it was caused by ignorance and misunderstanding. And so they responded with the compassion that they themselves never received. They worked hard to educate their community, to teach others about AIDS. In the end, Ryan wound up reaching far more than those in Kokomo, Indiana. He reached the entire nation.

The story of an ill young man who was kept out of school and shunned by his community wouldn't stay hidden in a small Midwestern town for long. Ryan's plight quickly became national news, and soon he was a household name. Ryan was on national talk shows and nightly news broadcasts. He was on the cover of *People* magazine. He was actually quite a shy boy, and Jeanne, a wonderfully unpretentious woman, certainly wanted no attention for herself. But the Whites felt it was their duty to speak out, to tell the world what they were experiencing. They wanted to make life better for thousands of others who were suffering in the same way – and not just other haemophiliacs who had contracted HIV but *everyone* living with the disease.

While bigots such as the famous preacher Jerry Falwell and the American politician Jesse Helms were spreading the hateful message that AIDS was a curse from God against gays, here was a dying teenager and his mother, thrust into the spotlight, standing shoulder-to-shoulder with *all* people living with HIV/AIDS. It was the height of bravery, the height of compassion. I love them for it to this day. By speaking out, Ryan and Jeanne helped to normalise the epidemic and relieve some of the terrible stigma and fear surrounding it. In doing so, they also hastened the government response and increased the urgency of medical research. What's more, they demonstrated what we now know to be the truth – that we must love all those living with HIV/AIDS if we are ever going to eradicate the disease itself.

Like millions of people, when I read about Ryan in that magazine, sitting in the doctor's waiting room, I was incensed. More than that, I was overcome with the desire to do something for him and his family. 'This situation is outrageous,' I thought. 'I've got to help these people.'

As angry and motivated as I was, I hadn't a clue what I could do for them. I suppose I was thinking that I would help raise awareness about what the White family was going through, or perhaps raise money to fight AIDS. But how could I help others when I couldn't help myself?

The truth is, I was a huge cocaine addict at the time. My life was up and down like a fucking yo-yo. My sense of values was buried under my self-destruction. I was still a good person, a kind person, underneath – otherwise I would have never reached out to the Whites in the first place. All I hoped was that somehow I could bring this boy and his family some comfort and support.

It turned out, in the end, the Whites would do far more for me than I ever did for them.

In the spring of 1986, after Ryan won his right to return to school, he and Jeanne came to New York to attend a fund-raiser for AIDS research and to appear on *Good Morning America*. I saw their interview, and I called Jeanne the next morning. I wanted to meet Ryan. I wanted to help. I invited Ryan and his family to one of my concerts.

Ryan was too sick to attend the first concert I planned to bring him to, but eventually I was able to fly the Whites to Los Angeles. They came to two of my shows, and then I took the family to Disneyland, where I had arranged a private tour and a party for Ryan. I wanted to give him an adventure – limos, planes, fancy hotels – a carefree time to take his mind off his pain and his difficult circumstances. But what I remember most about that visit is that I had at least as much fun as Ryan, if not more.

I felt instantly comfortable with the Whites, instantly

connected to Ryan. While we came from different countries, we really were cut from the same cloth. The Whites
were commonsense, straight-shooting people. They
were caring and humble and always grateful. What I
did for them on that trip, and subsequently, was out of
the pure love I had for this family. And that's really
what it was: love. I fell in love with the Whites right
away.

Getting to know the family put into stark relief what
a terrible mess I was. You can't imagine how selfish I
was at the time, what an asshole I had become. It was
partly the drugs, partly the lifestyle I had created, partly
the people around me, who indulged my worst instincts.
I had everything in the world – wealth, fame, *everything*
– but I'd throw a fit if I didn't like the curtains in my
hotel room. That's how upside down I was. That's how
pathetic I had become.

Ryan, on the other hand, was dying. His family had
been tormented. And yet, during his trip to L.A. and
every time I was with him from then on, he was relentlessly upbeat. At Disneyland, Ryan was so weak that I
had to push him around in a wheelchair for part of the
time. For a child, being wheelchair-bound at Disneyland
must be incredibly frustrating, not to be able to run
around and play at one of the world's largest play-
grounds. But Ryan loved every minute of it. He loved

life. Ryan wasn't thinking about dying; he was thinking about living, and he was getting on with it. His time was too precious to feel sorry for himself. I was with Ryan quite a lot over the years, and I can't remember a single time when he complained about anything. I know he wasn't a perfect child; there's no such thing. But Ryan was special.

So are his mum and sister. Jeanne was going through the most torturous episode any parent could imagine: watching her child die a slow and painful death, and not being able to do anything about it. But she never asked, 'Why me?' She embodied forgiveness and acceptance and perseverance at every turn, even though she must have suffered greatly in her most private moments.

Andrea was just like Jeanne; you couldn't get her down, and you never heard her complain. The youngest in the family often gets all the attention, especially someone like Andrea, a beautiful teenage girl, an athlete, a wonderful student. But Andrea's life took a backseat to Ryan's illness. She had to give up competitive roller-skating, her passion, for financial reasons. Like Ryan, she lost friends and was teased. She had it very rough. I was amazed by how she dealt with the reality of her family's situation with maturity and wisdom well beyond her years.

This family inspired me in a way that I cannot fully

explain. Being around the Whites touched me at my very core. I guess you could put it this way: I wanted to be like them. I wanted to be part of their family. They made me want to change, to be a better person, to be the person I knew I was on the inside. But this wasn't an easy thing to do, because of my addictions, because of my lifestyle. I was beginning to open my eyes to reality, but it took Ryan's death to open them completely. When his eyes closed, mine opened. They've been open ever since.

After the Whites came to L.A., from then on, I did whatever I could for them. Little things, mostly. Ryan came to more concerts. I sent gifts and flowers and cards. I called to check in. In 1987 Jeanne decided to move the family to Cicero, Indiana, a small town outside Indianapolis. She knew it was the right thing to do after Ryan confided in her that he didn't want to be buried in Kokomo. They needed to escape the place that had caused them such grief – that much was clear. One day, Jeanne called. With a great deal of hesitation in her voice, she asked if I might loan her part of the down payment she needed for her new home in Cicero.

To that point, Jeanne had never asked for a single thing. That she was now coming to me for help meant she badly needed it. I knew how desperate she was to give Ryan and Andrea a better life, so I told her to forget about a loan, I would simply send her the money. But Jeanne absolutely *insisted* on a loan. In fact, she made both of us sign a home-made contract stating that she would pay me back! Sure enough, years later, I received a cheque from Jeanne. I put the money straight into a college savings account for Andrea. Jeanne resisted, of course, but I told her that I *wanted* to help, that it meant something to me to support her family in this way. Looking back on it, I think she was being more charitable in continuing to accept my assistance than I was being supportive in giving it.

The Whites had a completely different life in their new home in Cicero. They were welcomed with open arms. Ryan did have a few friends in Kokomo, but in Cicero he became something of a local hero. The Whites were not only accepted but embraced, and Ryan thrived in his new school, making the honour roll as well as making many good friends.

It's not the case that the residents of Cicero were better or kinder human beings than the residents of Kokomo. My own opinion is that people are more or less the same all around the world; and besides, these two towns are only thirty miles apart. In fact, people in Cicero had many of the same questions, and shared many of the same fears, as people in Kokomo. Was it safe for the other children to be around Ryan? Did he pose a health risk to the community? The difference was that Cicero knew more about HIV/AIDS by the time Ryan arrived.

For one thing, Ryan had done much to educate the entire nation. Everyone knew his story, and in learning about Ryan's plight, America learned about AIDS as well. In addition, Ryan's new school held extensive AIDS education classes for the entire student body as well as the staff. The school board even sponsored conferences for parents and other members of the community to learn about AIDS, all before Ryan ever set foot in the classroom. He also had a champion and a wonderful friend in Jill Stewart, the president of the school student body, who happened to live down the street from the Whites.

Thanks to Jill's efforts, and the community's, Ryan's classmates were compassionate toward him, not fearful. Parents understood that their children weren't at risk, and they were able to ease any concerns among Ryan's classmates. Some children even taught their nervous parents about the disease. In the end, people weren't afraid; they were supportive. Cicero was able to see beyond Ryan's illness and focus on the amazing person he was.

Ryan found a bit of peace in Cicero, though not from his disease. He never wanted to give up – that goes without saying – but his fragile body had endured too much. In the spring of 1990, toward the end of his junior year of high school, Ryan was hospitalized with a severe respiratory infection. Jeanne called to tell me that Ryan was on life support. I immediately flew to Indiana. NFL star Howie Long and actresses Judith Light and Jessica Hahn were on the same US Airways flight. They had befriended Ryan and taken up his cause as well.

I spent the last week of Ryan's life by his hospital bedside, supporting Jeanne and Andrea in any way I could. Mostly that meant playing the family receptionist, and I was honoured to do it. Many people were trying to reach Ryan by phone and by mail – friends, celebrities, politicians, everyone wanted to express their support. Ryan was in and out of consciousness, but he was awake when Michael Jackson called. Michael was the biggest star in the world at the time, perhaps the most famous man on the planet. Years earlier, he had befriended Ryan as well, and one of Ryan's prized possessions was a red Ford Mustang that was a generous gift from him. As Ryan lay dying, he was so weak that he couldn't speak to Michael. I held the phone to his ear as Michael offered him kind words of comfort and love.

I grew very close to Jeanne during the final week of

Ryan's life. She described me then as her guardian angel, since I was able to help the family during this terrible moment by handling logistical details, and by simply being there for them. But it was the other way around. Jeanne and her family were guardian angels to me. And the message they were sent to deliver was very clear: it might be my deathbed next.

I had all the money in the world, but it didn't matter, because I didn't have my health. I wasn't well. But unlike Ryan, a cure existed for my substance abuse, for my self-destructiveness. As I stood next to Ryan's hospital bed, holding Jeanne's hand, seeing his bloated and disfigured body, the message was received. I didn't want to die.

As it happened, on the evening of 7 April, I was scheduled to play a massive concert in Indianapolis, not far from Riley Hospital for Children, where Ryan was being treated. The show was called Farm Aid IV, the fourth in a series of concerts meant to raise awareness and donations for family farmers in America. Months earlier, I had happily agreed to join Garth Brooks, Guns N' Roses, Neil Young, Jackson Browne, Willie Nelson, John Mellencamp, and many other amazing performers to put on this show. But at that moment, with Ryan near death, I didn't want to leave his side.

I rushed to the Hoosier Dome and hurried onstage. Other performers were in their usual stage dress, but I was wearing a baseball cap and a Windbreaker. I was so upset that I didn't care what I looked like, and it showed. Even 60,000 screaming fans couldn't chase away the grief I felt then. Since there were many musicians, each of us performed only a few songs. I started with 'Daniel' and then played 'I'm Still Standing.' Before my third song, I told the crowd, 'This one's for Ryan.' They burst into applause. The news of Ryan's hospitalization was a national story, and everyone knew he didn't have long to live. I played 'Candle in the Wind,' and the response was overwhelming. I looked out into the crowd, and people were holding up their lighters, thousands of little vigils flickering in the darkness for my dying friend.

When I finished the song, I ran offstage and rushed back to the hospital, back to Ryan's bedside. That's where I was, hours later, when Ryan died on the morning of 8 April 1990.

I'll never forget the funeral. I'll never forget the numbness of tragedy. I'll never forget what he looked like in the open casket, or the drive from the service to the cemetery. It was raining. We drove very slowly, in both grief and caution. I'll never forget Jeanne thanking me, in the middle of the greatest loss of her life, taking the time to acknowledge my being there with her. How surreal it all felt, like an awful dream.

It was the end of a very long week. It was the end of a very long fight.

Jeanne had asked me to be a pallbearer and to sing a song at Ryan's funeral. I wasn't sure that I would be able to keep my composure, but I agreed to do the song. I couldn't say no to her, but I didn't know what to sing. I didn't know what would be appropriate for such a tragic and painful occasion.

I ended up going back to my very first album, *Empty Sky*, and to the song 'Skyline Pigeon,' which Bernie Taupin and I wrote together. It's always been one of my favorites, and I thought it was the best track on that first album, maybe even the best track we had written to that point. It's a song about freedom and release, and it seemed fitting for Ryan's funeral. Now that he had passed away, I figured that Ryan was free to go wherever he wanted, his soul was free to travel, his spirit was free to inspire people around the world. I decided I couldn't be alone on that stage, though, so I taught the choir from Ryan's high school to sing along with me.

There was a picture of Ryan on the piano in front of me, his casket behind me. I hardly ever sing that song any more. My godson died several years ago, when he was only four years old. I played 'Skyline Pigeon' at his funeral, too.

There were more than 1,500 people in attendance at Ryan's funeral – not only his family and friends but celebrities he had touched and dignitaries of the highest order. Michael Jackson was there. Judith was there. Howie and Phil Donahue were among my fellow pall-bearers. First Lady Barbara Bush was there, too. Everyone was overcome with grief, even those who barely knew Ryan.

Some people from Kokomo attended the funeral as well, including the lawyer for the parents' group that had tried to block Ryan from attending school. He offered his condolences to Jeanne and asked her to forgive the way their town had treated Ryan. She did, without a moment's hesitation.

Over the course of the year following his death, Ryan's gravesite was vandalized four times. The poor child couldn't even rest in peace. Still, Ryan's message lived on. On the base of his tombstone, seven words are inscribed: patience, tolerance, faith, love, forgiveness, wisdom, and spirit.

I loved my friend Ryan more than I can express. I loved that he didn't have an ounce of quit in his heart. I loved that he didn't have a speck of self-pity in his soul. It wasn't just the way he held his head high as he struggled with not one but two terrible diseases. It wasn't just the way he bravely confronted death at an age when most children have no clue how precious life really is. No, Ryan was a true hero, a true Christian, because he unconditionally forgave those who made him suffer.

It's easy to think that Ryan's time on earth was hell. But he never saw it that way. He loved being alive. He loved the simple pleasures of friends and family. He lived his short and painful life with total grace and, above all, total forgiveness. In living the way he did, and in dying the way he did, Ryan changed the world. And he changed *my* world.

There's a scene in *The Lion King* where Rafiki, a wise and trusted elder, tells Simba, the hero of the movie, that he can bring Simba to see his deceased father. Rafiki leads Simba to a pool of water. At first, Simba sees only his own reflection. But then, the image of Simba's father appears in the pool. Rafiki tells Simba, 'He lives in you.' When I was writing and recording songs for *The Lion King*, that scene always reminded me of Ryan, and it still does, all these years later.

Ryan lives in me. Ryan and his family helped me to see the meaning of dignity, the importance of self-respect, the power of compassion. I'm here today because of Ryan. He inspired me to fix my life and to start my AIDS foundation. He continues to inspire me each and every day. I know that he looked up to me, and the thought of disappointing him now, even though he is long gone, makes me shudder. I try to honour his memory by living the way he would want me to live, by being the person he thought that I was.

Our friendship was the catalyst that helped to change my life. Indeed, Ryan *saved* my life. But mine is only one of countless lives that were saved by Ryan White.

Two years before he died, Ryan testified before the President's Commission on AIDS, which was a committee formed by the Reagan administration to investigate the epidemic and provide policy recommendations to the White House. Ryan and Jeanne travelled to Washington, and Ryan, only sixteen years old at the time, bravely told his story and greatly impressed the commission. Just weeks after Ryan died, Jeanne travelled back to Washington and exhibited extraordinary bravery of her own. Still reeling from the loss of her son, she personally lobbied members of Congress to dramatically increase funding for AIDS research, treatment, and education.

In August 1990, only four months after Ryan's death, Congress passed the Ryan White Comprehensive AIDS Resources Emergency (CARE) Act in his honour. The bill, which was approved with overwhelming and bi-partisan support, more than doubled government spending to combat the AIDS epidemic. Today, over twenty years later, Ryan's law provides more than $2 billion in AIDS treatment and prevention services each year to half a million Americans. The vast majority of those who receive assistance through the Ryan White CARE Act are low-income, uninsured people living with HIV/AIDS. In other words, the law embodies what Ryan taught me, and what he taught us all – that we must show compassion for everyone. Only then will we win the fight against this terrible disease.

In casual conversation with HIV/AIDS professionals, you often hear, 'This program is funded by Ryan White.' Of course, they are referring to the law. But the law exists because of the person, my friend. That Ryan's name is spoken by hundreds, maybe thousands, of people each day is an incredible testament to the impact of his life and legacy.

Ryan White's candle burned out long ago, but his legend never will.

2

A Decade of Loss

Ryan was not the first friend I lost to AIDS, and he was not the last. So many have been taken from me by this disease – sixty, seventy, eighty, I honestly don't know how many. I'd rather not count. But I never want to forget them.

That's why I have a chapel in my home in Windsor, in an old orangery on the property. It's where I go to remember the people in my life who touched me, who made me the person I am today. When I go inside it's like stepping back in time. I'm flooded with sadness and warmth.

Pictures adorn the walls. My grandmother. Princess Diana. Gianni Versace. Guy Babylon, the amazing keyboard player I lost to a heart attack in 2009. Then there's another wall, full of plaques that list name after name after name. People who, in my memory, are frozen in time as young, vibrant, and full of life. None of them are here any more. They all died of AIDS.

These were close friends, lovers, and people who worked for me. Many of them died in the 1980s, wiped out by a cruel and relentless plague. The first person I knew who died of AIDS was my manager's assistant, Neil Carter. He was a lovely young man, and I was distraught when I learned he had the disease. Three weeks later, he was dead. His was the first plaque I placed in my chapel.

Today, AIDS in the West is increasingly thought of as just another chronic condition that can be controlled with medication. We see people like Magic Johnson living long and healthy lives, and we wouldn't know they had such a terrible disease unless they told us. Thank heaven for that.

But when you got AIDS in the '80s, you died – quickly and horribly.

Imagine your mouth filling up with so many sores that you cannot eat. Your lungs filling up with so much fluid that you cannot breathe. A fatigue so crushing that you cannot lift your head off the pillow. Losing control of your bladder, your bowels, your mind. This is how my friends died in the '80s. It's how millions continue to die around the world.

I will never, ever forget being in those hospital rooms, seeing the hollow, devastated look in the eyes of friends who were racked by pain and by the knowledge that only death would end their suffering.

The physical depredations of AIDS were bad enough. Then there was the terrible indignity that AIDS visited on the infected: the shame and the stigma.

In the West, we often recall the madness and the misinformation, the suffering and the hopelessness of AIDS in the '80s as a sad but thankfully closed chapter in history. For much of the world, however, this chapter continues. In many parts of Africa, Asia, Latin America, and the Caribbean, AIDS is every bit the death sentence, every bit the scarlet letter, that it was for a New Yorker or San Franciscan who contracted the disease in 1982. It's a similar story among poor and low-income people in Western countries – more so than we like to admit. When I think back on the '80s and recoil at the horror of that time, it infuriates me that history is repeating itself right now, all over the world.

Today, even though AIDS is a top killer worldwide, it's often an afterthought among the public and in the press. Back in the '80s, though, as Ryan's story vividly illustrates, the outbreak of AIDS was greeted by a level of public hysteria that was unprecedented in modern history. And because the earliest reported infections were among gay people, intravenous drug users, and Haitian immigrants in the United States, it was all too easy for society to scapegoat and scorn them. Of course, there were plenty of heroic advocates for people living with HIV/AIDS back then. But very early on, there were far too many in the media, religious institutions, governments, and the general public who sent an unmistakable message to people with AIDS: We do not care about you.

I can't imagine any worse treatment for a human being. To have people believe they are completely on their own, that they must struggle without a loving touch or a kind word, is one of the cruellest things you can subject another to, no matter the illness or the situation. That's precisely what happened to thousands of people with AIDS in the '80s. They were rejected by their families and ostracised by their communities. They were made to feel that they had somehow brought the disease upon themselves through their own sinfulness or lack of virtue.

I'm deeply ashamed that I didn't do more about AIDS back then. My friends were dying all around me, and with few exceptions I failed to act. I gave some money to foundations. I performed at AIDS benefits. I helped the Whites. I recorded a song called 'That's What Friends Are For' with Gladys Knight, Stevie Wonder, and Dionne Warwick; the proceeds from that single went to the American Foundation for AIDS Research, or amfAR. But the fact is that I was a gay man in the '80s who didn't march. I didn't give the time or effort that I easily could have, and should have, to fight AIDS and support those who had it.

Instead, I was consumed by cocaine, booze, and who knows what else. I apparently never got the memo that the 'Me' Decade ended in 1979. The Elton ego train kept rolling right through the '80s. I spent most of that time as a passive bystander to this human calamity that was unfolding all around me. I was very conscious of AIDS. I knew what it was. I knew it was killing my friends. I just didn't have the strength or sobriety to do anything about it.

I don't remember the first time I heard the word 'AIDS.' Perhaps that's because the disease began its rampage across the globe a few years before it even had a formal name. But I do remember hearing about gays falling ill of some strange disease as early as 1982. There were hushed whispers at parties and rumours in the air. A palpable fear took root in the gay community long before it consumed the general public. I also remember that my earliest understanding of and inter-action with AIDS occurred in America. America is where I often lived and worked. It's where the disease first emerged as an epidemic. And it's where the fate and future of AIDS would be decided by America's powerful government, media, and research institutions.

Although no one knew its significance at the time,

the first official reporting of the AIDS epidemic was on 5 June 1981, when a weekly CDC bulletin noted a strange outbreak of a rare pneumonia in five gay men in Los Angeles.[1] A month later, reports surfaced of a rare cancer called Kaposi's sarcoma appearing in forty-one homosexuals in New York and California. These were initially presumed to be isolated outbreaks, and no one knew exactly what was causing them.

It was only later that researchers realized these rare pneumonias and cancers were connected.

A select few cancer doctors and epidemiologists realised something serious was afoot from the word go. But among the public, the media, and most policy makers, few were paying attention to these outbreaks that seemed to affect only urban gays on the coasts.

When you go back and read the news stories from 1981, however, it is absolutely eerie. In hindsight, there was clearly a gathering storm of the epidemic to come. In a 3 July 1981 *New York Times* story on the Kaposi's sarcoma outbreak, reporter Lawrence Altman described most cases involving 'homosexual men who have had multiple and frequent sexual encounters with different partners.' Most had also used drugs. Altman said researchers allowed for the possibility that a virus could have caused the outbreak, but they thought it seemed unlikely. After all, cancer isn't contagious. Altman noted

34

toward the end of the article, however, that the patients seemed to have severely compromised immune systems, as evidenced by 'serious malfunctions' of 'T and B cell lymphocytes.'[2]

What Altman described – the sex, the drug use, and most important the compromised immune systems and T-cell damage – would soon be recognized as the defining risk factors and characteristics of AIDS. But until then, these strange outbreaks would be known as peculiar afflictions of the gay community. In fact, as outbreaks popped up in new cities, they were often described as 'gay cancer' or 'gay pneumonia.' Once researchers realised that these diseases and other strange opportunistic infections that were emerging in otherwise healthy gay men were connected, they began calling it Gay-Related Immune Deficiency, or GRID.

But that didn't last long. By 1982, heterosexual injection drug users were getting sick. Soon, the disease showed up in the infant children of infected mothers. And there was a notable cluster of the disease among people of Haitian descent in Miami and New York. Some medical professionals were calling it the '4H disease,' named for the four groups thought to be at highest risk of infection: homosexuals, haemophiliacs, heroin users, and Haitians. Then, in August 1982, the CDC coined the name that would stick, a name that would soon cause panic around America and the world: Acquired Immune Deficiency Syndrome.

For a while, to the extent the epidemic was considered at all, it was considered an affliction of 'them' – the queers, the junkies, the immigrants, those people we don't like to think about or talk about. But AIDS became a disease of 'us' the moment rumours hit that it was in the general blood supply. First, AIDS began showing up in people with haemophilia, like Ryan. The real panic took off when patients started contracting the disease from blood transfusions during surgery, and although the numbers would ultimately turn out to be relatively small, the public began to feel as if anyone could get the disease. 'Fear of AIDS Infects the Nation,' blared a *U.S. News & World Report* headline at the time.[3]

Fear of AIDS in the blood supply was completely understandable; it was based on facts. But the worst public fear about AIDS was that you could contract it just from casual contact with an infected person. This was, of course, utter nonsense. You can't get HIV from a toilet seat or a swimming pool, from mosquitoes, by hugging someone with AIDS, or by breathing the same air in a room with someone who is HIV-positive. Blood and sexual fluids are, and have always been, the *only* transmission routes for HIV. Period.

As I've said, this was well understood very shortly

after the epidemic was discovered. By early 1983, scientists had not identified precisely what virus was causing AIDS, but they knew for certain that casual contact did not transmit it. Some public health organisations, including the CDC, did what they could to get the facts out, but they were overwhelmed by a tide of misinformation, often from people and organisations that should have known better. On 6 May 1983, the *Journal of the American Medical Association* published a news release with the headline 'Evidence Suggests Household Contact May Transmit AIDS.'[4] As late as 1985, a White House lawyer who is now the chief justice of the U.S. Supreme Court, John Roberts, sent a memo to President Reagan saying, 'There is much to commend the view that we should assume AIDS can be transmitted through casual or routine contact.'[5]

With these mixed signals coming from high-ranking government officials and the medical establishment, it's no wonder that people indulged in irrational fears. In New York, the state Funeral Directors Association recommended that its members refuse to embalm people who had died of AIDS.[6] In Louisiana, the state house of representatives overwhelmingly passed a measure permitting the arrest and quarantine of any person with AIDS (the law was thankfully revoked soon thereafter).[7] In San Francisco, when a local TV station tried to tape a special to increase public understanding of AIDS, the studio technicians refused to let people living with HIV/AIDS onto the set.[8]

Across the country, reports began to emerge of targeted persecution and violence against people with HIV/AIDS, particularly gays. In Seattle, one group of young men rampaged through a local gay district, beating people with baseball bats and raping two men with a crowbar. When one of the attackers was arrested, he told police, 'If we don't kill these fags, they'll kill us with their fucking AIDS disease.'[9]

Calming this rampant hysteria required a forceful response from the American government, the only institution big enough, powerful enough, and knowledgeable enough about AIDS to make a difference. But the sad truth about AIDS in the '80s is that President Ronald Reagan, his administration, and many leaders in Congress refused to engage in the fight. They exhibited neither the urgency nor the focus that the crisis required. We needed a plan to kill this monster. We needed real money to fund research, treatment, and education. Most of all, we needed leaders who cared.

The AIDS epidemic flared and raged in the '90s because no one put it out when it was smouldering in the '80s.

The indifference started at the very top. President

Reagan did not publicly utter the word 'AIDS' until 1985, four years and some 13,000 cases into the epidemic. He did not give a speech on AIDS until 1987. Perhaps no one better catalogued the pattern of official indifference and apathy than the journalist Randy Shilts, whose 1987 book, *And the Band Played On*, remains the definitive investigation of what did and – more important – what did not happen during the early years of the AIDS epidemic. His book is full of stories, some of which I've recounted here, of frantic researchers and doctors on the front lines of the AIDS fight, begging their superiors, the Reagan administration, and Congress for more resources and attention to combat the disease. They were repeatedly ignored. Shilts himself died of AIDS in 1994.

In public, many administration leaders were sounding the right notes, as Shilts documents in his book. Margaret Heckler, for example, the secretary of Health and Human Services (HHS), spoke before the U.S. Conference of Mayors in June 1983. She pointedly told the crowd, 'Nothing I will say is more important than this: that the Department of Health and Human Services considers AIDS its number-one health priority.'[10] But behind the scenes, Heckler's very own people were contradicting what she said in public. A month after she told Congress the AIDS fight was fully funded,

Dr Edward Brandt, the assistant secretary for health at HHS, wrote in an internal memo that 'it has now reached the point where important AIDS work cannot be undertaken because of the lack of available resources.' He said that critical prevention programmes had been 'postponed, delayed or severely curtailed.'[11]

Over at the CDC, Don Francis, an epidemiologist leading the organisation's AIDS research, was far more blunt. In a letter to the director of the Center for Infectious Diseases, he wrote, 'The number of people already killed [by AIDS] is large and all indications are that this disease will not stop until thousands of Americans have died . . . Our government's response to this disaster has been far too little.'[12] At the time, for a government scientist to say as much was extraordinarily brave. Dr Francis and others like him were true heroes in their efforts to get their superiors, and the country, to wake up.

It's not as if the Reagan administration and Congress were incapable of responding forcefully to public health crises. As Shilts noted, in October 1982, when seven people in Chicago were killed by cyanide-laced Tylenol, federal, state, and local officials mobilized all the manpower and money necessary to figure out what had happened and to develop procedures to ensure it didn't happen again.[13] There was a similar all-hands-on-deck attitude years earlier when a rare pneumonia, later named Legionnaires' disease, struck and killed thirty-four people at a July 1976 American Legion convention in Philadelphia.[14] And yet AIDS – an epidemic that was killing thousands of Americans and people around the world by the mid-'80s – didn't even warrant enough attention for the president of the United States to utter its name in public.

The charitable explanation for the official inaction on AIDS is that decision makers just didn't know how bad it really was. If you were a doctor seeing AIDS patients every day, a CDC epidemiologist tracking the geometric spread of the disease, or a gay man living in New York's Greenwich Village or the Castro neighbourhood in San Francisco, you could see that this was something new and terrible. You knew the only chance to beat the disease was to channel the same urgency and attention you'd give to something your life depended on. Because it very much did. We needed what one prominent AIDS researcher called 'a minor moon shot.'[15] But for many in government, perhaps AIDS felt like a distant, vague threat. Everyone knew someone with cancer or diabetes. In the early 1980s, however, most people didn't know anyone with AIDS.

I think that people are fundamentally good, which is why I *want* to believe the primary reason that AIDS did not receive the attention it deserved was due to ignorance – that people just didn't know. But, in my heart, I know this isn't true. I've lived too long and seen too much to accept that AIDS was ignored because we didn't understand the danger of the disease. AIDS was ignored because too few people in power cared about those who had it.

At a congressional hearing in 1982, California congressman Henry Waxman, one of the earliest champions for people with HIV/AIDS, described what I still believe to be the core truth about the epidemic:

> This horrible disease afflicts members of one of the nation's most stigmatized and discriminated-against minorities. The victims are not typical, Main Street Americans. They are gays, mainly from New York, Los Angeles and San Francisco. There is no doubt in my mind that, if the same disease had appeared among Americans of Norwegian descent, or among tennis players, rather than gay males, the responses of both the government and the medical community would've been different.[16]

Of course, we'd soon discover that AIDS was not a gay disease at all. It was a disease that could cut down anyone, anywhere. But AIDS would continue to carry that early gay stigma throughout the 1980s, and for many religious and governmental leaders, that was all the excuse they needed to turn their backs and blame it all on a community they already loathed. Even to this day, AIDS remains a disease closely associated with the gay community.

It still stings to recall the pure, unadulterated hatred that was spewed at gays and AIDS sufferers. Jerry Falwell, the founder of the Moral Majority and a key ally of President Reagan, said that 'homosexuals are violating the laws of nature. God establishes all of nature's laws. When a person ignores these laws there is a price to pay.'[17] Pat Buchanan, the former Nixon speechwriter and future presidential candidate, echoed that sentiment when he was quoted as saying, 'The poor homosexuals – they have declared war upon nature, and now nature is exacting an awful retribution.'[18]

You couldn't help but detect a touch of glee in these statements. People such as Falwell had been preaching for years that the Lord would condemn America for its sinful ways. And here, finally, was a righteous God inflicting a plague on those faggots who had been flouting His divine laws. It was truly sickening. And if you think this hatred was purely the domain of funda-mentalist preachers and combative commentators, consider what happened in Texas in 1985. That's where the state health commissioner, Dr Robert Bernstein, proposed that AIDS patients be quarantined from the general public.[19] It's where the former mayor of Houston, Louie Welch, said one way to curb the AIDS epidemic would be to 'shoot the queers.'[20]

I know that these awful bigots weren't representative of their constituencies, or everyone in the church or in government. Not even close. And didn't we all stop paying attention to the fire-breathing preachers when they blamed the gays for 9/11 and Hurricane Katrina? Good grief. But in the 1980s, these people had real power. Jerry Falwell's Moral Majority helped put President Reagan in the White House in 1980. He delivered the benediction at Reagan's renomination at the Republican convention in 1984. The man had *major* influence. He could have used it to heal. If he'd managed a more thorough reading of the Bible, perhaps he would have noted the part where Jesus heals the leper who had been shunned by everyone else.

But Falwell and his ilk used their power to incite hatred. Their horrifying words and inaction gave people license to ignore the suffering of those with HIV/AIDS. They contributed to the general sense that AIDS was not a national or a global problem but a gay problem, a drug-addict problem, an urban problem. And by doing so, they helped guarantee the AIDS epidemic would get far worse.

In 1985, as the situation was indeed worsening, two things happened that significantly changed the perception and trajectory of the AIDS epidemic.

French and American researchers had finally identified the virus that caused AIDS by 1984, and although there was a dispute over the credit for discovering the virus and what it should be called, it would eventually become known as the human immunodeficiency virus, or HIV. But it wasn't until March 1985 that the U.S. Food and Drug Administration (FDA) approved the first-ever blood test to screen for HIV. The test was relatively crude, and it was initially used only to screen donated blood. But it was something. Scientists finally knew what was causing AIDS, which gave desperate patients some small hope that this would eventually lead to a treatment.

That wouldn't come until 1987. Until then, doctors couldn't do much for AIDS patients other than help manage the symptoms. This forced many of those living with HIV/AIDS to turn to a variety of strange, experimental, and mostly useless treatments. I remember friends flying to Mexico to get amino acid injections. Adopting radical nutritional regimens. Taking all kinds of off-label drugs used to treat illnesses such as cancer or metal poisoning, with the hope that these would somehow, someway have an effect on their disease. These people, every single one of them, would be disappointed. There would be no miracle cure coming. But that first HIV test laid the groundwork for a revolution in the way scientists and doctors treated and researched AIDS.

Then, later in 1985, a second announcement revolutionized the way the American public saw the disease: Rock Hudson, one of the most famous leading men in the history of Hollywood, announced that he was dying of AIDS. When the news first hit over the summer, the public wasn't told exactly how Hudson had become HIV-positive. People close to Hudson speculated he might have got the virus from a blood transfusion during heart surgery.[21] But everyone in Hollywood, and in the circles I ran in, knew that Rock was gay and that he had in all probability contracted the disease sexually.

The media attention was absolutely insane. People simply could not believe that this strapping, six-foot-five-inch movie star, this paragon of the alpha American male, had AIDS. By the time Hudson died on 2 October 1985, the secret of his sexuality was out, but somewhat to my surprise, this didn't seem to turn the public against him. Instead, I remember hearing a lot about Rock Hudson being the new 'face of AIDS' and comments like 'If Rock Hudson can get it, anyone can get it.'

I've always found it deeply ironic that after four years of gay men dying of AIDS, a turning point in Americans' perception of the disease was . . . a gay man dying of AIDS. But Rock Hudson didn't fit prevailing stereotypes of homosexuality. He was the ladies' man who starred in *Pillow Talk* with Doris Day. He was a close friend of Ronald and Nancy Reagan. Rock became the 'respectable' face of AIDS, and perhaps AIDS itself became a bit more respectable, a bit less vile, because he had it.

Hudson's death didn't miraculously end the apathy and the bigotry surrounding the disease, of course. Far from it. But it did help to change the way the public perceived people with AIDS, and it compelled the government to get more serious about the disease. Less than three weeks after Hudson died, the U.S. Senate appropriated $221 million for AIDS research, nearly twice the amount approved the year before. After Rock Hudson's death, ignoring AIDS was no longer an option. The perception of AIDS was changing. So was the reach of the disease itself. By 1985, AIDS had been discovered throughout the globe. It was a true pandemic.

Although powerful institutions such as the U.S. government and the media had finally begun to recognise AIDS for the public health crisis that it was, fear and ignorance would continue to cloud the response. Many of the people who had been indifferent to the disease early on became pure hysterics in the late 1980s, peddling hare-brained ideas to tame the epidemic. Conservative icon William F. Buckley suggested tattooing everyone with AIDS. He wanted to brand the forearm of IV drug users and the buttocks of homosexuals.[22] The more 'respectable' version of Buckley's scarlet lettering called for mandatory HIV testing of all gays and other 'high risk' individuals. Never mind that HIV tests in the '80s often gave false positives. Or that mandatory testing would drive the very people who needed to be in the medical system away from it. Or that virtually every major public health official considered the idea idiotic. Mandatory testing was the type of simple, straightforward idea you could sell to a public that was justifiably frightened of a disease they still didn't quite understand, because their government was doing little to educate them about it, let alone fight it.

The idea of mandatory testing was surprisingly discredited by, of all people, C. Everett Koop, Ronald Reagan's arch-conservative surgeon general. Known mostly to the public for his anti-abortion views, Koop's 1986 report on AIDS was a revelation. The report didn't just dismiss mandatory testing as impractical and counter-productive. It called for AIDS education at 'the earliest grade possible' and for the widespread distribution of condoms.[23] This was heady stuff. Five years into the epidemic, the surgeon general's report represented the first major governmental effort to educate the public about AIDS. The fundamentalists were furious at Koop's frank discussion of the disease and the sexual behaviour that spread it, but to his credit, he stood by his findings. (It's interesting to note as a point of comparison that, a year earlier, the British government had distributed information about HIV/AIDS to every single household in the UK)

In 1987, President Reagan finally gave a speech on AIDS. It was, in many ways, an underwhelming speech, filled with platitudes and too few commitments to action. But finally the president said what the nation needed to hear: 'It's also important that America not reject those who have the disease, but care for them with dignity and kindness . . . This is a battle against disease, not against our fellow Americans.'[24] We could have used those words in 1982, but they were better late than never.

As the Reagan administration was waking up from its long AIDS slumber, the scientific fight against the disease was moving forward as well. In March 1987, the first treatment to slow the progression of AIDS was approved by the FDA. The drug, AZT, was an anti-retroviral that had proven in clinical trials to delay the onset of AIDS in HIV-positive patients. Patients who received AZT treatment remained HIV-positive – the drug wasn't a cure – but it allowed them to live a bit longer with the virus. The drug was adding a few months or years to patients' lives. And it often had awful side-effects. In fact, the symptoms caused by AZT were sometimes worse than those of the disease itself. The anaemia was crippling; it caused haemophiliac-like symptoms. Some people were taken off the drug because it was too toxic, but often, doing so would cause a spike in AIDS symptoms. It was a horrible way to survive. I remember some of my friends taking AZT and suffering terrible nausea and vomiting. A few developed anaemia. But after years of utter despair, this drug was a ray of hope. It was something to slow the disease down, and it promised more treatments to come.

For many, however, AZT would come too late to make a difference. That was tragically the case for Ryan White, as it was for one of my very closest friends, a man whom I loved dearly, and a man who was loved by millions of people around the world: Freddie Mercury.

Freddie didn't announce publicly that he had AIDS until the day before he died in 1991. Although he was flamboyant onstage – an electric front man on a par with Bowie and Jagger – he was an intensely private man offstage. But Freddie told me he had AIDS soon after he was diagnosed in 1987. I was devastated. I'd seen what the disease had done to so many of my other friends. I knew exactly what it was going to do to Freddie. As did he. He knew death, agonizing death, was coming. But Freddie was incredibly courageous. He kept up appearances, he kept performing with Queen, and he kept being the funny, outrageous, and profoundly generous person he had always been.

As Freddie deteriorated in the late 1980s and early '90s, it was almost too much to bear. It broke my heart to see this absolute light unto the world ravaged by AIDS. By the end, his body was covered with Kaposi's sarcoma lesions. He was almost blind. He was too weak to even stand.

By all rights, Freddie should have spent those final days concerned only with his own comfort. But that wasn't who he was. He truly lived for others. Freddie had passed on 24 November 1991, and weeks after the funeral, I was still grieving. On Christmas Day, I learned that Freddie had left me one final testament to his selflessness. I was moping about when a friend unexpectedly showed up at my door and handed me something wrapped in a pillowcase. I opened it up, and inside was a painting by one of my favorite artists, the British painter Henry Scott Tuke. And there was a note from Freddie. Years before, Freddie and I had developed pet names for each other, our drag-queen alter egos. I was Sharon, and he was Melina. Freddie's note read, 'Dear Sharon, thought you'd like this. Love, Melina. Happy Christmas.'

I was overcome, forty-four years old at the time, crying like a child. Here was this beautiful man, dying from AIDS, and in his final days, he had somehow managed to find me a lovely Christmas present. As sad as that moment was, it's often the one I think about when I remember Freddie, because it captures the character of the man. In death, he reminded me of what made him so special in life.

Freddie touched me in a way few people ever have, and his brave, private struggle with AIDS is something that inspires me to this day. But his illness, I'm ashamed to admit, wasn't enough to spur me to greater action. I've railed against government and religious leaders who were indifferent to or who actively undermined the fight against AIDS. They deserve every bit of criticism I'm throwing their way. They could have done so much more.

I could have done so much more, too.

As I said, I was appallingly absent from the early

fight against AIDS. With large swathes of the government asleep at the switch, grassroots activists led the way. Everyday Americans such as Larry Kramer, who simply would not go away, who would not shut up about the crisis in their communities. People like Elizabeth Glaser, the great advocate for paediatric AIDS research, whose determination forced people in power to pay attention to AIDS. But the most famous, and one of the very first to stand up for those living with HIV/AIDS, was my dear friend Elizabeth Taylor.

Elizabeth was the brightest star in Hollywood, one of the biggest celebrities in the world. Everyone knew her as beautiful and classy and elegant, and she was most certainly all those things. But she was also willing to get her hands dirty. She was willing to stand up for gay people when few others would. She was willing to get into the nitty-gritty of AIDS policy and to fight for the cause, without a moment's hesitation or thought for her own reputation.

When Rock Hudson announced he had AIDS, Elizabeth stood by his side and stood up for him in public. As early as 1986, she was testifying before Congress, urging more funding for emergency AIDS research. And Elizabeth helped to take the AIDS fight global, speaking in 1989 at an AIDS benefit in Thailand, the first event of its kind in South-east Asia. Many people even credit Elizabeth for personally convincing President Reagan to speak publicly about AIDS in 1987. Perhaps most important, she lent her support to Dr Mathilde Krim, who, with Elizabeth's assistance, built amfAR into a world-class organisation focused on HIV/AIDS biomedical research. To this day, it is one of the foremost AIDS organisations in the world.

Another wonderful friend who helped change the public perception of AIDS was Princess Diana. Diana and I were very close, not only in our friendship but in our world-views. Indeed, our relationship stemmed from the fact that we shared the same values, the same sense of humour, the same love of people and connecting with them. Diana was one of the most compassionate people I've ever known, and she used her tremendous pulpit to communicate the power of love and understanding.

When it came to the AIDS epidemic, like Elizabeth, Diana was among the first global figures to speak out. She did more than that, in fact. She reached out, quite literally, to those living with HIV/AIDS. In 1987, Diana opened the first hospital AIDS ward in Britain. Reports of her shaking hands with AIDS patients raced around the globe, and a big deal was made of the fact that she was not wearing gloves. At the time, many were still frightened to have any contact whatsoever with someone living with HIV/AIDS. Diana, with a simple yet profoundly human gesture, helped to ease the hysteria and correct the harmful misinformation surrounding the disease.

In the years that followed, Diana continued to raise awareness about the AIDS crisis, and pictures of her touching and interacting with HIV-positive people went a long way to calm irrational fears that continued to persist. In fact, she never stopped championing those living with HIV/AIDS. In 1997, just before her tragic death, Diana and I had been in discussions about her taking on an active role with my foundation as global ambassador for our work. She met with my staff, and we were all thrilled at the prospect of working together. Had she not been taken from us so soon, I know she would have continued to greatly impact the fight against AIDS.

Princess Diana, Elizabeth Taylor, Elizabeth Glaser, Mathilde Krim, Larry Kramer – these are my heroes, among many others. They worked hard and they accomplished much when it mattered most. I should have been by their side, following their example. Today, all I can do is follow in their footsteps. But back then, in the '80s, I could have made an impact early in the fight, just like them. I was a huge star. I had lots of money. I had powerful friends. And I was gay.

I sometimes like to joke that I'm the acceptable face of homosexuality, a blokey, non-threatening type, someone your mother wouldn't mind having over for dinner. If I had been a more committed advocate for people living with HIV/AIDS in the '80s, maybe I could have diminished, just a bit, the stigma or the suffering of some poor gay man in San Francisco or Dallas or Dublin. Maybe not. But at least I could have tried.

Instead, I spent the '80s sinking ever deeper into a drug addiction that began in 1974, when I was recording my album *Caribou* in Colorado. Even though I'd been a fully fledged rock star for years by then, I still hardly even knew what cocaine was. I was unbelievably naive. I remember walking to the back of the studio one day, seeing a line of white powder on the table, and asking my manager, 'What on earth is that?' He told me it was cocaine. I figured I'd take a little sniff.

I knew some people who could casually do cocaine once a month. I was not one of those people. By the 1980s, I was completely hooked on coke, booze, and eventually food. Then I became bulimic, too. I was guilty of every single one of the seven deadly sins, except sloth. No matter how bad it got, I never lost my work ethic or my love of music.

But I had become numb to everything else. I had friends dying left and right of AIDS. I would go to the funerals. I would cry. I would mourn, sometimes for weeks on end. None of this changed my behaviour. In fact, it just got worse. I was doing more drugs to block out the horror of it all. I was sleeping around without protection, drastically increasing the chances I would contract the very same disease that was killing the people closest to me. It's no small miracle that I never contracted HIV myself.

I was extremely selfish and self-destructive. I could barely hold myself together, let alone be out there with the Elizabeth Taylors of the world as an AIDS advocate.

It took Ryan's death to wake me up, to transform my life.

3

Starting Over

I returned to London after Ryan's funeral and locked myself away at home, as had become customary, even before his death. I had reached the point where I didn't know how to speak to someone unless I had a nose full of cocaine and a stomach full of liquor. And increasingly even that wasn't enough.

I remember watching television a few days after the funeral; they were running a tribute to Ryan, playing a recap of the funeral service. There I sat, watching myself on-screen at one of the lowest points of my life. I looked horrible. My hair was white, my skin pale. I was bloated and gorged. I looked tired and sick and beaten down. Seeing myself that way, at Ryan's funeral, was almost too much to take. I had been overcome by addiction; I was completely out of control. I looked, quite frankly, like a piano-playing Elvis Presley. As messed up as I've ever been. There was no question: I was going to change, or I was going to die. Even while spiralling, I knew that much was true.

And I desperately *wanted* to change. I remember many days when I would just sit there, alone in my room, drinking, using, bingeing, listening to Peter Gabriel and Kate Bush sing 'Don't Give Up' on repeat.

In this proud land we grew up strong
We were wanted all along
I was taught to fight, taught to win
I never thought I could fail
No fight left or so it seems
I am a man whose dreams have all deserted
I've changed my face, I've changed my name
But no one wants you when you lose.

'No one wants you when you lose.' That line always got me. I would listen to those lyrics, and then it would get to the chorus – 'Don't give up,' they would sing, and I would weep at the thought. I didn't want to give up, but I was falling farther down the rabbit hole with every gram of cocaine. I would think, 'I'll get well one day. I will. I will. I hate this life. I hate me. I hate what I've become.' But I couldn't – or, I should say, wouldn't – ask for help.

Everybody tried to get me to stop. And I appreciate

that enormously now, I really do. But at the time it infuriated me. Many people in my life back then had to suffer through my rage, my denial, my refusal to listen. I knew I was an asshole. I knew I had a problem. But I believed, wrongly, very wrongly, that I was intelligent enough and wealthy enough and famous enough that I could get control all by myself. Of course, the more I thought that, the worse I got.

Some people call it a 'high bottom.' It's what happens when you hit rock bottom, but you aren't actually in the gutter. That's where I was. I was successful. I was rich. I had a boyfriend at the time, Hugh Williams, who loved me dearly, and I loved him. I had the respect and admiration of strangers. It was the life I had always wanted – or, at least, something approximating it. 'How could I have hit rock bottom,' a voice in the back of my head would say, 'when I'm on top of the world?'

But I had. The drugs had taken over my life. So had the alcohol. And the food. My self-obsession had morphed into an incredibly low self-image. I could no longer control anything. Not how I acted, or what I took, or what I ate. About the only thing I could control was whether I kept it down. So in addition to bingeing on coke and booze and food, I was purging. Then I'd rinse and repeat. I was an addict. I was bulimic. And everything was getting worse. Each day, I would think about how much I wanted to change. But each day, the disappointment that I hadn't changed drove me to use more. It was a bitter, bitter cycle.

I was reminded of Ryan constantly, of how disappointed he would be in me, alive and capable of doing plenty of good in the world but instead choosing to satisfy my worst urges at every opportunity. To this day, I am relieved beyond words that he never knew that side of me. I don't want to imagine what the weight of his disappointment would feel like. Better to think of how proud I know he would be if he could see how much I've changed. And how much he changed me.

Weeks passed, and things didn't get any better. Then one day – I remember it like it was yesterday – Hugh told me he was going to rehab. He didn't want to be a drug addict any more, he said. He didn't want to live this life any more. He needed help and he couldn't do it himself. Looking back, I should have been proud of him for the sheer bravery of that decision. I should have supported him. Of course, I didn't. I was furious.

I should say that I had, and on occasion still have, a terrible temper. It was made worse by the fact that I was in a very bad place, that Hugh calling himself a drug addict might as well have been him calling me one. And though I *was* one, how dare he say so! I said some horrible things to Hugh – things I would forget saying if I could, things that no one should have to hear. It wasn't enough, thank goodness, to stop him. Hugh left for rehab that day. I, on the other hand, retreated further into my addictions.

I withdrew to my house in London and used solidly for a week. Locked in a room with my cocaine and my own stubbornness. The truth was, as much as I tried to convince myself that Hugh had betrayed *me* – that he had left *me* alone, that it was *his* fault, that *he* was wrong – I knew how ridiculous that was. I was the true culprit. Besides, I loved Hugh very much, and I missed him terribly. I was alone with my addictions, my self-pity, my self-loathing. You really can't be more alone than that.

One day, somehow, I worked up the courage to try to find Hugh. I got in touch with his ex-boyfriend Barron Segar, who is now on the board of the Elton John AIDS Foundation (funny how things work out), and he was able to track Hugh down at a halfway house in Prescott, Arizona.

I still remember how nervous I was when I called him. I thought he might hate me for the things I had said, the way I had acted. He should have. I wouldn't have blamed him for it. What made matters worse is that I knew he was in recovery, and he probably wouldn't want to associate with someone who was still using.

That's one of the things they tell you. You can't be around that sort of thing. And 'that sort of thing' was me. Still, I had to give it a try.

My fingers trembled as I dialled the phone number. And then, there he was, finally, on the other end of the line. I told him I wanted to come see him, that I needed to. 'Listen,' he said, 'you can come to see me, but you need to speak to my counsellor on the phone first. There are some things I want to say to you that need to be said. I'll have a counsellor and you'll have a counsellor and we'll sit and we'll talk.'

I agreed. 'Whatever it takes,' I thought. I called up Hugh's counsellor, who told me that it was fine for me to visit, but before I did, I needed to write down the three things I disliked most about Hugh. And he would be doing the same. We would sit down face-to-face and discuss our lists.

I knew what was about to happen. It was going to be some kind of intervention. There was a time, not long before that phone call, when I would have simply hung up. But this time was different. I knew this needed to happen, whatever it would be, however it would unfold.

Later that week, I flew to Arizona. I arrived at the hotel in Prescott and went up to the room. I knocked on the door and waited with intense anxiety for someone to answer. The door opened, and there he was. There was Hugh. He looked absolutely terrified to see me. The two counsellors were there, too. Hugh invited me in and introduced me to them. One of them asked me to sit directly across from Hugh and told me that through all of it we needed to look each other in the eye. I was told to go first; I was to read my list of three things I didn't like about Hugh.

'You're untidy,' I said. 'You don't put the CD back in the case when you're done with it. And you leave the lights on when you leave a room.' That was my list. That was all I could come up with.

Then it was Hugh's turn. He pulled his paper out of his pocket, and I could see that he had written a full page. I can't remember everything he said, but I'll never forget this part: 'You're a drug addict. You're an alcoholic. You're a food addict. You're bulimic. You're a sex addict. And you're codependent.' His voice was quivering while he said it. He must have been terrified of how I would react. Knowing my temper, he must have thought I was going to tell him to fuck off. 'How dare you talk to me like that!' he must have thought I would say.

But I stayed silent. I sat there and I took it. I was scared, too. I was shaking as much as he was. But I kept saying to myself, 'You've got to stay here and you've got to hear this. You've got to hear the truth.'

'You need to get help,' Hugh said. That was the last thing on his page, and then there was silence. It was my turn to respond. It was the pivot point of my entire existence, right there in that hotel room in Prescott. I had a choice, and what came next honestly changed my life forever.

'You're right,' I said through tears. 'You're right. I'll go somewhere. I'll get help.'

In that moment, my soul came alive again. I could feel it. It's a strange thing to say, but it was as if my pilot light came back on. Instead of fear, I felt relief. Instead of anxiety, I felt calm. It was as if Ryan were sending me a message, letting me know it was going to be okay. I've learned that you have to listen to those messages when they're being sent, just like the message I received standing by Ryan's deathbed just two months prior. This time, I was ready. I was ready to change.

Immediately, I was on the phone with my doctor. If I was going to go to treatment, it was going to happen right away, and on my terms. But that would be its own challenge. It turned out that, at the time, there weren't many places that treated men for eating disorders. Back then, men were thought to account for about 10 per cent of people with such disorders. It just wasn't considered a real problem. What made matters harder was that there were even fewer rehab facilities that were willing to treat multiple problems at once. Dual diagnosis was discouraged, for reasons I still do not agree with. Most treatment centres expected you to go to one facility to be treated for your eating disorder before you went to another for your drug addiction, and then yet another for alcoholism. That wasn't acceptable to me. I felt very strongly at the time (and I still do) that all of my problems had the same root cause, and that I couldn't treat one without treating them all. Luckily, we found a place in Chicago that would take me in and treat all my addictions at once: Parkside Lutheran Hospital.

Less than three months after Ryan died, I was on a plane to Chicago, determined to change my life. I entered rehab in July of 1990, and I am incredibly proud to say that I have been sober ever since.

My time at Parkside Lutheran was as challenging as it was transformative. The first days were especially difficult. When you deprive your body of cocaine after having used very much and very frequently, as I had, the craving for it is inconceivably enormous. I went through bouts of extreme anxiety and irritability. I couldn't sleep. I couldn't think about anything but my own misery. This was compounded by the fact that I had stopped using not just cocaine but everything I had self-medicated with: the booze, the food, the sex.

I was depressed and alone. I felt sick and weak and foggy. Needless to say, the first stages of rehab were among the most trying periods of my life.

The most important part of my time in rehab was that, to all with whom I interacted, I was not Elton John the rock star. I was just Elton. Elton the addict. For years I had thought that my station in life provided me with the tools I would need to help myself. I thought I was somehow uniquely situated to overcome what other people could not. How wrong I was.

From the moment I walked into that hospital, the playing field was levelled. We were all the same. Suffering, struggling addicts who wanted to get better but didn't know if we could. We were all people who had made bad choices and seen the consequences, but then made the same choices despite ourselves. And we had done so again, and again, and again. The truth of it all was that simple: no matter where we had come from, what we had accomplished or failed to accomplish, what our life experiences had been up to that point, we were all the same. And none of us would get better without asking others for help.

The path to recovery wasn't a straight one, by any means. I remember quite clearly, on many occasions, wanting desperately to run away. Two separate times, I came awfully close to doing just that. It didn't merely seem like the easier path; it categorically was. I could have left, been on a plane back to London, and been back in my room, with the relief that would come with the buzz of cocaine and a drink. If not for Ryan and Hugh, I would indeed have run away.

Thank God I stayed. Over time it did get easier. I could feel a genuine transformation happening inside me. I was working hard at it, and I could feel myself changing. Every day of staying sober was a challenge, but it was invigorating to feel that I was regaining control over my life, my direction, my choices. And I'd say the biggest driver of my progress was the overwhelming kindness of the strangers I met in rehab.

People were remarkably helpful. They seemed willing to do anything for me, even though they didn't know me. They talked to me, they encouraged me, they listened to me. I still get emotional when I think of all the friends I met there, people who would come up and spend time with me during a meeting, after a meeting. They would phone me to check in. I was surrounded by innumerable acts of human kindness. It brought me back to life, I really believe it did. Enormous empathy. Enormous compassion. And because it was coming from people who had gone through what I had, who were just like me, it was easy to accept their embrace. Before rehab, I would say to those who tried to help me, 'What do you know? You don't understand.' But these people, they understood. They really understood. It didn't matter what their religion was or their political party or their background. That never, ever came into it. They were just helping their fellow man. And I was lucky that man was me.

There was an incredible dignity in the process, an extraordinary amount of humanity, and to feel that way when I was most vulnerable was unexpected and welcome. I talked a lot. But mostly I listened. And I spent a long time on my recovery, sometimes kicking and screaming along the way. But I did as I was told. I took the help and direction of others. And it worked. No one can alter his or her behaviour instantaneously. You can't change overnight. And yet you *can* change. It is possible. But it requires learning to become a human being again first.

Six weeks after I entered the programme, I was released. It was September 1990. I returned to London. There were a lot of people who wanted to see me take the stage immediately, to get on with the life I had left behind while in rehab. I chose, instead, to take an entire year off. Recovery, I was told, and have since learned, is a long process. It doesn't end after six weeks. It doesn't end when you leave the hospital. It never ends. It takes constant, hard work. For the first time in my life, I would dedicate myself to my own betterment. When I returned to my career, I wanted to return truly transformed. This was, after all, a second chance I hadn't deserved. In Ryan's memory, I could not afford to squander it.

4

Starting Up

Several months after returning to London, I decided to relocate to Atlanta. I wanted to be back in America, a country that had been very good to me, but I felt I ought to avoid Los Angeles and New York, where temptation might well get the better of me. During this time, the first thing I wanted was to continue to get well. And the second thing I wanted – just as badly as the first, really – was to give back.

In sobriety, I was constantly reminded of the good I could have been doing to help those with HIV/AIDS – my friends, people like them, people like me – but how little I had actually done. There were many potential acts of selflessness that I chose to forgo in exchange for another line or another drink. I had been lucky to emerge from the '80s without having contracted HIV myself. And I was even luckier to have emerged from treatment healthy, able to do something meaningful with my life. I owed a lot to many people – Ryan,

Jeanne, Andrea, Hugh – but to that point, I simply had not delivered. It was time to do something about that.

The first step was, literally, a small one, but it was inspirational. Hugh was in Atlanta with me, and he and I participated in AIDS Walk Atlanta. This was the city's first AIDS walk, I believe, and there were thousands of people who came out to participate. I was very glad to be one of them. Raising awareness is a critical aspect of the fight against AIDS today, and it was even more so in 1990. The mass of people taking to the street made quite an impression – on me and on the public – and I was thrilled to stand up and to be counted that day. I was also incredibly moved. There I was, in the street, surrounded by people who had been directly impacted by the AIDS epidemic. Some of those I walked with were HIV-positive. Or, like me, they had friends or family members who had died of AIDS. For the outside world, the AIDS Walk put a human face to the epidemic. For me, it crystallized the need to get more personally involved.

Soon after, I started volunteering for a wonderful organisation in Atlanta called Project Open Hand, a charity that arranged the delivery of home-cooked meals to AIDS patients all over Atlanta. My dear friend John Scott and I would drive around the city and deliver meals to home-bound people who were very sick. I'll never forget the tragedy we witnessed doing this work. The stigma at the time was punishing. If you had AIDS, you were ostracised by most of society, period, just as Ryan had been shunned by his community in Kokomo. In Atlanta, and all over America, people were contracting HIV and then losing their jobs, their insurance, their friends; even their own families would turn away. People with HIV/AIDS were on their own in every sense. And the sicker they got, the more difficult it was for them to leave the house. The stigma associated with the disease was so intense that if someone with full-blown AIDS had a medical emergency and needed to go to the hospital – as people invariably did in the early 1990s before effective treatment was available – some emergency personnel refused to assist AIDS patients. The people to whom we were delivering meals were literally shut out of the world, and as a result far too many became shut up in their homes – a retreat not of choice but of unjust circumstance.

There was something about volunteering that reminded me of the strangers I had met while in treatment. To the people we were visiting, I wasn't a celebrity. Some must have recognized me, and I do remember a few startled looks as I walked through the door with a hot meal. But to most, I was just a rare friendly face, coming for a brief social interaction, offering a meal and what little comfort came with it. It was also a reminder of just how hard things were for people dying of AIDS – a recognition that it wasn't just the disease but society's response to the disease that had taken a toll. There were some people John and I delivered meals to who opened their doors and were happy to greet us. There were others who cracked their doors just wide enough to take what we were offering, give a quick thanks, and shut themselves back in. And, sadly, there were still more who had completely closed themselves off to the world that had betrayed them. For these poor souls, we just left the meal on the front porch. We would ring the doorbell, but no one would answer.

I imagine that everyone I ever delivered a meal to is dead. I am still haunted by the thought of how many good, innocent people suffered horrible deaths completely alone in those years.

In volunteering for Project Open Hand, John and I were making a small difference. But I wanted to do more. I *had* to do more. People were dying. People like *me* – gay men, addicts or those in recovery, my friends, and my friends' friends. It was an atrocity, and I wasn't going to sit idle any longer.

John and I soon got involved with other organisations in the city. We learned of the Grady Ponce De Leon HIV Center in Atlanta, a facility that aimed to identify all of the existing opportunities for someone who was suffering from HIV, whether it was indigent care, critical care, or other social services. The programme helped people with everything from finding a doctor to applying for unemployment insurance after losing a job. I was honoured to cut the ribbon to open the Center and raise awareness that this amazing resource was available to the Atlanta AIDS community.

And then, in October of 1992, Elizabeth Taylor asked me to join her for a benefit concert at Madison Square Garden to raise money for HIV/AIDS research. As I said, Elizabeth had been a trail-blazer in the fight against AIDS, and she was one of my closest friends. I immediately agreed. It turned out to be a beautiful event, and we raised a lot of money for the cause. It was also the final catalyst for one of the most important decisions I have ever made in my life – the decision to start a foundation devoted to fighting AIDS.

Several things in the lead-up to the benefit concert and then in its aftermath had struck me. First, it was clear that you could leverage fame and celebrity not only to raise a considerable amount of money but to raise awareness, too, something that was critical to breaking down the stigma that had grown up viciously around the AIDS epidemic. But second, as effective and important as individual benefit concerts were, the process felt piecemeal to me. When someone like Elizabeth Taylor mobilised the troops, we were, of course, happy to answer the call. And the money raised at such events went directly to fighting the disease. But there was something missing: a general lack of co-ordination. A single place where the money could be pooled and spent strategically would be more efficient and more effective. That way, I thought, we could maximise the bang for our proverbial buck.

It also struck me that the majority of the money being raised and spent in the fight against AIDS was getting directed toward a search for treatment and hopefully a cure. There's no question that, given the U.S. government's initial denial and then modest funding for research, this should have been the priority – and amfAR was doing an amazing job of filling the void. Especially then, in the early 1990s, we were convinced that the greatest hope for a cure lay in the minds of research scientists in labs around the world.

But there were other aspects of the disease that seemed, to a large degree, underfunded and overlooked: helping people protect themselves from HIV in the first place and helping HIV-positive people live better and die with dignity. That meant more than new drugs, which, again, were essential. It also meant transportation to the hospital or the pharmacy to get medicine. It meant access to doctors and nutrition and counselling. It meant education and programmes for prevention. It meant teaching people the importance of condoms, about how the disease is transmitted and, most important, how it isn't. It meant efforts to eliminate stigma and discrimination, and it meant medical, legal, and housing support for highly marginalised populations, those who were suffering the most but who had been pushed aside by a society that preferred to ignore reality rather than confront it. It meant, ultimately, recognising that people were forced to suffer as much emotionally as they were physically. All of this had to change.

As I had these epiphanies, a few days after Elizabeth's concert, the idea took shape in my mind. I called John. 'I'm starting an AIDS foundation,' I said, 'and I want you to run it.' John agreed, and two months later the Elton John AIDS Foundation – EJAF – opened its doors.

Or, I should say, 'door.' The door to John's home, that is. You might think that a celebrity foundation would have fancy offices and chauffeurs and a cappuccino maker. But we didn't have anything like that, and we still don't. Besides, celebrity foundations in 1992 were rare and, apart from Elizabeth Taylor's foundation, did not focus on AIDS. No one was really doing anything like that back then. So we improvised. John ran the organisation for two years from his breakfast table in

Atlanta. Virginia Banks, who worked on my team in Los Angeles, became the foundation's secretary and John's right hand. I asked Sarah McMullen, my publicist, to do double duty, working both as my PR guru and also as the foundation's fund-raiser. Thankfully, she agreed. And that was it. Just the four of us and an amazing board of directors. To this day, we continue to run the foundation with a skeleton crew.

When we started out, we didn't have any experience or infrastructure at all, only the feeling of absolute urgency, the sense that no amount of effort was sufficient. And it wasn't just our sense; it was the reality of the epidemic in those days. You cannot quantify the magnitude of human suffering – physical and psychological – the disease caused back then. So there was no time to lose. EJAF was created as an emergency response. And I had no inkling that the foundation would still be needed two decades later. As bad as things were in 1992, many of us thought that a cure was on the horizon, that some brilliant scientist would master the virus's code so that we could destroy it, that we would be able to close up shop and declare victory within a few years. Twenty years have now passed, and those hopes seem heart-wrenchingly naive. The barriers to a cure were far greater than any of us could have known at the time.

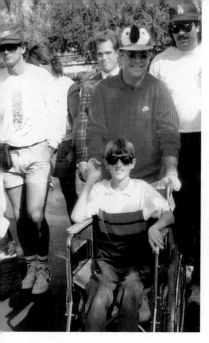

With Ryan White, a young boy who contracted HIV through treatment for hemophilia, at Disneyland in October 1986. Upon first hearing Ryan's story, I reached out to the White family to offer my help. It turned out, in the end, the Whites would do far more for me than I ever did for them. *(Jeanne White-Ginder)*

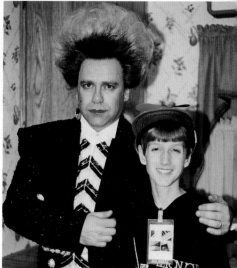

Ryan White and I first met backstage at a concert held in Oakland, California, on October 3, 1986.
(Jeanne White-Ginder)

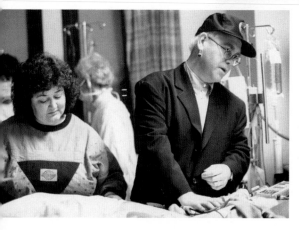

With Ryan's mother, Jeanne White, at Ryan's bedside at James Whitcomb Riley Hospital in Indianapolis in 1990.
(Taro Yamasaki / Time & Life Pictures / Getty Images)

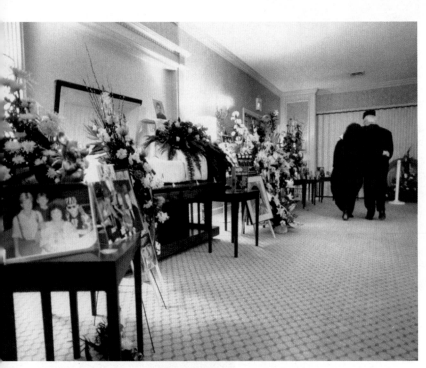

Embracing Jeanne as we grieve at Ryan's funeral.
Ryan passed away on April 8, 1990.
(Taro Yamasaki / Time & Life Pictures / Getty Images)

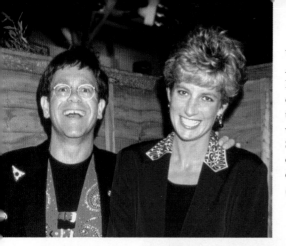

With my friend and fellow AIDS activist Princess Diana, backstage at a concert in 1993. Diana opened the first hospital AIDS ward in Britain in 1987. She was one of the most compassionate people I've ever known.
(Richard Young)

With Freddie Mercury, front man of the band Queen and one of my closest friends, at the Live Aid concert in London in July 1985. Freddie was diagnosed with AIDS two years later. He passed away on November 24, 1991.
(Rex USA)

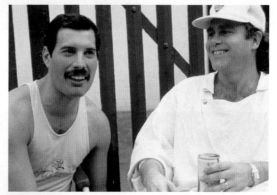

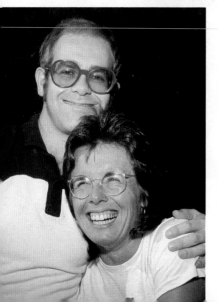

With my dear friend Billie Jean King in 1975. Billie Jean and her partner, Ilana Kloss, had the idea for "Smash Hits," an event that would bring tennis stars together for an EJAF fund-raising event built around exhibition matches. We've held Smash Hits every year since 1993, and it's grown to be one of our most important and successful fund-raisers each year.
(James Fortune / Rex / Rex USA)

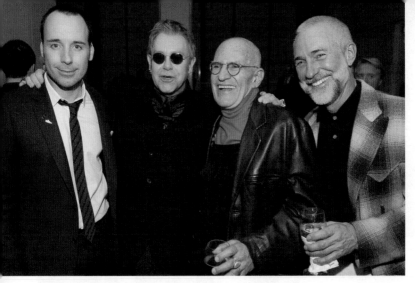

With my partner and EJAF chairman David Furnish, Larry Kramer, and David Webster at "amfAR and ACRIA Honor Herb Ritts" in New York City. Larry Kramer, who cofounded the Gay Men's Health Crisis in 1982, is one of my heroes in the fight against AIDS. *(Dimitrios Kambouris / WireImage / Getty Images)*

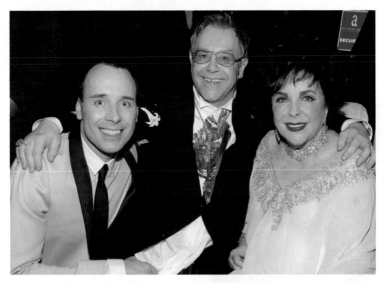

David, Elizabeth Taylor, and I attend EJAF's thirteenth annual Academy Awards Viewing Party. A longtime AIDS activist, Elizabeth was the founding international chairman of amfAR, the American Foundation for AIDS Research. She was willing to stand up for gay people when few others would. *(KMazur / WireImage / Getty Images)*

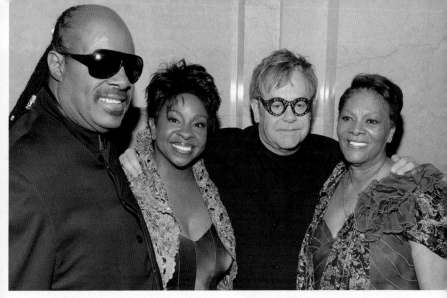

Stevie Wonder, Gladys Knight, Dionne Warwick, and I reunite backstage after singing "That's What Friends Are For" at the amfAR New York Gala on February 9, 2011. We originally recorded the song in 1985, with proceeds of more than $3 million going to support amfAR. *(Larry Busacca / Getty Images)*

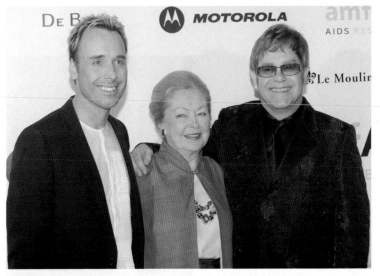

With David and Dr. Mathilde Krim at amfAR's Cinema Against AIDS 2002 benefit gala in France. Mathilde Krim is the founding chairman of amfAR. *(Evan Agostini / ImageDirect / Getty Images)*

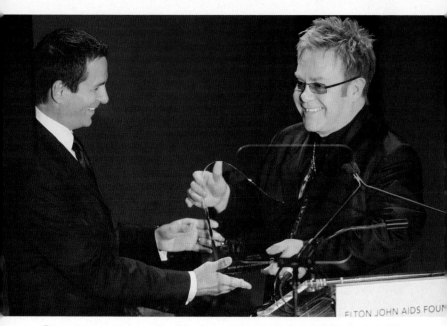

Presenting a special award to John Scott at the "An Enduring Vision" gala in New York, November 2, 2005. John was EJAF's first executive director. In the organisation's early days, his kitchen served as our makeshift office.

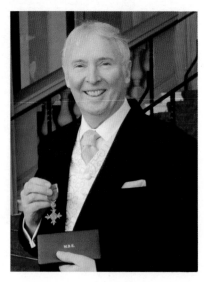

EJAF-UK executive director Robert Key at his MBE investiture for services to charity. Robert ran the foundation in the UK until he passed away in 2009.

(© Gerry Lane)

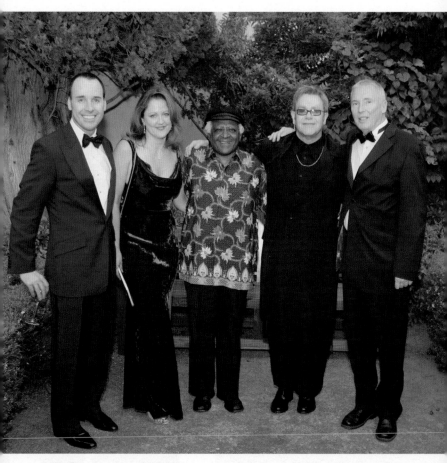

With David, current EJAF-UK executive director Anne Aslett, Desmond Tutu, and Robert Key at EJAF's fund-raising ball in Cape Town, South Africa, on January 8, 2005. *(Marc Hoberman)*

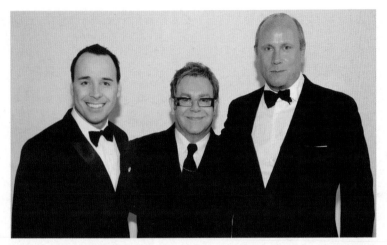

With David and EJAF executive director Scott Campbell at the National Association of Broadcasters Education Foundation gala on June 11, 2007. I was honoured to receive the Service to America Leadership Award. *(© Oscar Einzig)*

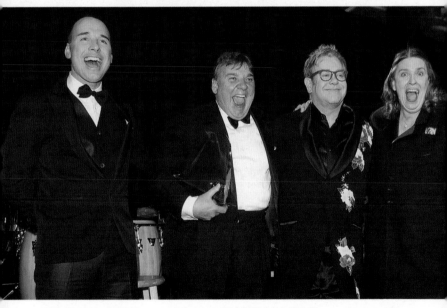

With David and EJAF trustees Johnny and Eddi Barbis at EJAF's seventh annual "An Enduring Vision" benefit, held in New York on November 11, 2008. EJAF honoured the couple that night with an Enduring Vision Award. *(Theo Wargo / WireImage / Getty Images)*

In formulating our response strategy, we asked two important questions: How would we define the foundation's mission? And how would we turn our ideas into action as swiftly as possible?

Strange as it may sound, the solutions were largely driven by the lessons I had learned in rehab. To get well, I had to confront the reality of my own life and change it. That required self-reflection. It required a willingness to be honest with myself. I felt that this confrontation with reality, this embrace of honesty, had to be part of how my foundation took on the epidemic. We had to face facts.

Of course, the realities of AIDS were – and are – very uncomfortable for many people. The disease exists in every population, but it is heavily concentrated in marginalised populations, in people society finds awfully easy to turn its back on: the gay community, sex workers, drug users, the impoverished and uneducated. If we were going to be honest about the disease, we needed to target populations that were suffering from it, regardless of how uncomfortable it might make people feel.

I wasn't going to shy away from that. Because, guess what? People do survive on the streets selling sex. People do use drugs. That won't change by our turning a blind eye to them. And I knew, from personal experience, that everyone deserves the same level of dignity and humanity.

After all, I was a recovering addict. Who was I to feel superior to anyone else? I didn't, and I still don't. The bottom line is, we're all human, and we all deserve to be helped and to be loved. I was determined to infuse my foundation with that set of values. To this day, what drives our work more than anything else is the idea that all people with HIV/AIDS deserve dignity and compassion.

I was also determined to have a hands-on relationship with our work. I wasn't interested in just lending my name to the cause, or performing a few songs on stage now and again. I had more to give than that. I wanted to give my ideas and my energy. I wanted to give my time. This was going to be a major priority in my life, I felt, just as important as my career.

To start off, we wanted to focus on the tremendous need for the basics – the real basics – food, lodging, transportation, medical attention, education, legal support, and counselling. These were the things that John and I had seen firsthand were lacking, the kinds of things we knew we could improve. The mission I decided on was to provide funding for such basic programmes, with the ultimate goal of reducing the incidence of HIV/AIDS, eliminating the stigma and discrimination associated with the disease, and providing direct treatment and care services to HIV-positive people, to allow them to live with dignity.

Within the first year, all of the critical elements had come together for the organisation. I covered the operating costs initially, so that every dollar we raised would go into services. But there was such an overwhelming need, we felt as if we could never – and would never – get the money out the door fast enough. Everything we did, every fund-raiser we held, every cheque we wrote, it all felt like one act of genuine desperation. We never even considered putting together a savings account. All we thought about was how to raise money, more and more money, and then get it into the right hands immediately. I know, looking back, that we were doing good work. But we were also witnessing such immense and wrenching suffering that I don't think any of us believed we were succeeding. I don't think you can ever really feel that way when so many people are dying.

Raising money, it turned out, was not the hardest part, thanks to the hard work of John, Virginia, Sarah, and our amazing board of directors. I had convinced many great friends from the music and entertainment industry to join our board to help get EJAF up and running: Robert Earl, the founder and CEO of Planet Hollywood and later the CEO of Hard Rock Cafe, and Art Levitt, the CEO of Hard Rock Cafe International; Howard Rose, my long-time agent; Al Teller and his right-hand man, Glen Lajeski, of MCA; Johnny Barbis, the music executive and my manager of many years; and Michele Burns, the former CEO of Mercer Consulting who, at the time, was a senior partner at Arthur Andersen. All of our original board members were serious businesspeople and also wonderfully caring friends of mine. They made the right connections for us and taught us how to run EJAF with the efficiency of a successful commercial enterprise like the ones they had built. They raised an extraordinary amount of money, and I'm so proud that several of them remain on our board to this day.

Many of these early board members helped us establish innovative ways of fund-raising, by using our celebrity and commercial connections to develop and market products that would be sold for the benefit of EJAF. It was amazing that heavy-hitting companies and people were willing to spend money for us this way. Barron Segar, a banking expert, helped devise a credit card that directed a percentage of expenditures to support the foundation's work. Billie Jean King and Ilana Kloss had the idea for 'Smash Hits,' an event that would bring tennis stars together for a fund-raising event built around exhibition matches. We've held Smash Hits every year since 1993, and it's grown to be one of our most important and successful fund-raisers each year. Eddi Barbis was instrumental in engaging and sustaining a long-term, cause-related marketing project. The photographer Herb Ritts, who sadly died of complications from AIDS himself, auctioned his amazing work to support EJAF. Whoopi Goldberg developed a T-shirt for us that was sold at Planet Hollywood, and Jane Fonda and Ted Turner lent their celebrity and efforts to our cause as well, giving the foundation a tremendous boost in both resources and credibility.

Over the years, we've partnered with many companies on a range of fund-raising products and activities, and it's been fantastic for all of us – the companies elevate their profiles while raising a ton of money for an important cause, and the foundation directs the proceeds to critical efforts. It's exciting to see that, today, so many other organisations have adopted this model.

So raising money was, in some ways, the easy part. The challenging part was, how do we distribute funds with lightning speed and in a strategic way at the same time? John and I didn't have the expertise to know which organisations in which cities or states needed our funding the most. But we knew that we had to figure it out, and we weren't going to waste a dime. One possibility was to create our own in-house grants process, whereby organisations around the country could apply for funding, and we could assess their relative merit. But there were problems with that model. The first, and most immediate, was that it would become quite expensive and labour-intensive to develop. We felt we didn't have time to do it, and we didn't want to sink funding into our own operations rather than pushing the money out the door to the people it was intended for. Beyond that, there was a sense that building our own grant-giving structure would be duplicative. There were other organisations that already had these structures in place. They could handle the distribution better than we could; we didn't need or want to re-invent the wheel. So, very early on, we made a key decision: our job would be to raise the money, and we would build partnerships to get it into the right hands. With the help of experts on our board, including Dr Charles Farthing and the incredible activist Eli Saleeby, this is how we would proceed.

We did an extensive search and were lucky – extraordinarily lucky – to find the National Community AIDS Partnership. The partnership was the brainchild of the Ford Foundation. To run their partnership, Ford hired an executive director, Paula Van Ness, who to this day is one of the most brilliant women I have ever met. What she understood in those early years was essential: with so many separate organisations providing their own services to their own regions, we needed some kind of nationwide model, something that would help us respond to the crisis in a truly co-ordinated and strategic way. We needed, for example, to get funding to places that had become epicentres of the disease – Los Angeles, New York, Atlanta. But we also needed to distribute funds in places like Tulsa, Oklahoma, where the number of AIDS patients was far fewer but where the suffering was just as great.

The goal of the partnership wasn't just to collect money and distribute it; it was to mobilise social service organisations that already existed, that already had infrastructure, and to turn their attention to HIV/AIDS. The National Community AIDS Partnership offered challenge grants to these organisations, and EJAF provided the funding. Organisations would get a grant, say, $10,000, with the requirement that they raise an additional $10,000 from their local communities. In this way, Paula worked with each organisation to develop independent, local fund-raising mechanisms. Thus, the partnership created AIDS treatment, care, and prevention start-ups all over the nation.

It was a terrific win-win situation for us and for the communities involved. There was no cost to EJAF in using the National Community AIDS Partnership's challenge grant distribution model. Nearly every single dollar we sent through the partnership was distributed to communities. And we weren't responsible for determining the most efficient use of that money. The local organisations knew their own critical needs; they got to decide where and how those funds would be distributed. EJAF's board would assess and approve each project we funded. On top of that, each dollar we spent through that process was matched at least two to one, if not three to one or more. The model was an extraordinary success, and it drove home an important early lesson that has stayed with us to this day: partnerships really do work, and replicating what others are doing is an absolute waste of money.

I will never forget the exhilaration and anxiety of those early days. I had the duelling senses that we were accomplishing great things but at the same time not accomplishing nearly enough. All we cared about was that people were dying, and we wanted to get them the care they needed and, at the very least, to enable them to live and die with dignity. It wasn't until a few years into the process that we really began to understand the kind of impact we were having. I clearly remember the day we received a report from the National Community AIDS Partnership that quantified our efforts. We had raised $1.5 million, and thanks to the challenge grant distribution model, we had generated $7 million in matching funds. Our model was working better than we could have ever imagined. We were moving the needle in a very real way.

By 1993, we had created a sister organisation in London dedicated to the same mission. As in the United States, we benefited immeasurably from a number of great friends who joined the board of directors of our fledgling UK foundation. Johnny Bergius was a prolific fund-raiser whose commitment to our cause led him to literally climb several mountains and journey to the North Pole in support of EJAF. Marguerite Littman, founder of the AIDS Crisis Trust, one of the first AIDS charities in the UK, lent us her expertise and ultimately integrated her charity into ours. James Locke, who has been living with HIV for almost thirty years, was an inspiration when we were starting out. Frank Presland, an old friend and legal genius, made fantastic contributions to our early efforts. Rafi Manoukian, the wonderful philanthropist, consistently helped us raise our sights in our global work.

Another UK board member was my dear friend Robert Key. Early on, I asked Robert to take on the job of running EJAF-UK. I had known him since the 1970s, when he started handling my record releases. I was thrilled that he agreed to take on the new role, and I knew he would be the perfect person to get our UK organisation off the ground. He was so personally committed to the cause that he initially refused a salary, though eventually the board forced him to accept one because of the amazing work he was doing. He ran the foundation until his untimely death in 2009.

The mission of EJAF-UK was the same as that of EJAF-U.S., but the mechanism was different. There was no UK equivalent of the National Community AIDS Partnership, and so Robert went out on his own and met with the various organisations that were working on HIV/AIDS treatment and prevention. He learned about the kinds of services they were providing for people living with HIV in London, but he also learned something else. It appeared that there was a burgeoning AIDS epidemic in Africa. The disease wasn't just a Western crisis. And so the UK arm of EJAF adopted a global focus. Robert, together with Anne Aslett, who now heads up the foundation, made EJAF-UK one of the first private foundations to have an explicit strategy in support of people living with HIV/AIDS in Africa and beyond. To this day, the UK office makes major investments to fund programmes in Europe, Africa, and Asia, while the U.S. office directs its grants to the Americas and the Caribbean.

None of this would have been possible without Robert. He was a force of nature. He made it his personal mission to learn everything about HIV/AIDS and what it was like to live with the disease. He wanted to understand what it felt like to experience the stigma and isolation, the opportunistic infections that would crop up, and the stress of knowing you could die at any moment. He spent time visiting hospitals, shelters, prisons, anywhere and everywhere, to meet and even nurse HIV-positive people of all ages and walks of life. Like Ryan, he bravely battled the stigma around AIDS with his own kindness, compassion, and love.

For the sixteen years that he ran my UK foundation, Robert saw firsthand what people living with the disease needed, and he used his experience to do some ground-breaking things such as ensuring the creation of a national HIV/AIDS Hardship Fund for people in poverty and pushing for higher standards of nutrition for AIDS patients. Thanks to him, EJAF was on the front lines of the UK's response to the African epidemic.

Robert's death was a blow to the AIDS community and a personal tragedy for me. He wasn't just a wonderful friend – he was one of the greatest crusaders against AIDS I have ever met.

There were many others who inspired me tremendously during those early years of my foundation. First and foremost among them is my partner of nearly twenty years, David Furnish, who is also chairman of the board of EJAF in both the United States and the United Kingdom.

David and I met in 1993, when I was still in the process of transforming my life and focusing on my recovery and my health. At the time, in addition to conquering the addictions that had imprisoned me for so long, I had purged many of the people around me who were enabling my destructive lifestyle in the first place. After completing my rehab and returning to London, I was looking for some new friends, and I was introduced to David at a dinner party I held one night.

But David would become so much more than a friend. We shared the same passions, the same sense of humour. We instantly connected, and we quickly fell in love. It's impossible to overstate David's impact on my life at that time, and ever since. He is there for me in every way imaginable. He focuses my energies in positive and productive ways. I would not be the man I am today if not for David. He was, is, and always will be the most important person in my life, alongside our son. We are partners in everything, including the work of EJAF. Together we were able to keep the foundation going, and growing, during its formative years.

Princess Diana was another source of inspiration to me, and as I mentioned, she had hoped to be a source of support to EJAF as well had her life not come to an end so tragically. Diana was always wonderfully encouraging, and not only about my AIDS work. Like David, she helped me keep my life on track during the first years of my recovery. I was sober and taking care of myself, but it wasn't always easy, and having the support of true friends like her was simply priceless.

One of my favourite memories of Diana was in 1993, when I went to battle with the *Sunday Mirror*, a British tabloid that had published a ludicrous story alleging I had lapsed back into bulimia and was seen eating and then spitting out my food at a party. Never mind that I was thousands of miles away when the party had taken place. I sued the paper for libel and eventually won. But one day, when the lawsuit was still under way, I received a letter in the mail. It was a handwritten note from Diana that read, 'Thank you on behalf of bulimics everywhere!' What a wit that woman had. She and I had bonded years before over our eating disorders, and she wasn't above poking a little fun at the seriousness of our struggles with food and with the press.

Like Diana, Elizabeth Taylor also kept us going with her example and her incredible sense of humour, and she supported my foundation in every way she could. Even as I grieved her recent passing, I was moved to learn that she had left a generous contribution to EJAF in her will, which speaks volumes about the tremendously caring woman she was.

But one story really says it all about Elizabeth. Ever

since EJAF was founded, we've put on a massive Academy Awards viewing party that serves as the biggest annual fund-raiser for EJAF-U.S. One year, despite being in horrible pain and very poor health, and on her birthday, no less, Elizabeth attended the event to help us raise awareness about HIV/AIDS, as she had done many times previously. There were dozens of photographers and reporters – perhaps more than a hundred, in fact – cramming the very long red carpet at the entrance to the fund-raiser. Elizabeth had a terrible time getting around at that point. But, with David on one arm and two of her grandsons on the other, Elizabeth walked the entire stretch. And not only that, she spoke to every single journalist and posed for every single camera that was aimed her way. More to the point, Elizabeth spent the whole time talking about the importance of EJAF's work and the urgency of the AIDS epidemic. She never once strayed from that topic. Elizabeth must have been on her feet for an hour, and the whole time she was as energetic and graceful as ever. Finally, when she reached the end of the red carpet and finished her last interview, Elizabeth turned her beautiful smile to David and whispered into his ear, 'Get me my fucking wheelchair!'

I miss my friends Elizabeth, Diana, and Robert more than you can imagine, and every single day. I think about them constantly, and EJAF would not be here but for their herculean efforts, inspiration, and support. With their help and David's – and thanks to John, our small but dedicated staff, and our wonderful board of directors – within only a few years, we were becoming a major player in the fight to rid the world of AIDS. There was much work to be done, huge mountains to climb. But, wherever he was, I hoped with all my heart that another dear and departed friend, Ryan, was proud. Indeed, I felt a sense of pride in myself as well. I was sober. I was giving back. I was alive. For the first time in years, I was really, truly, alive.

5

A Crisis of Caring

From this vantage point, looking back on it all, it's amazing to think how much has changed in the twenty years since I started the foundation. It's also amazing to reflect on how much remains the same.

For one thing, given the scope of the AIDS crisis today, we still operate with a sense of urgency, with the attitude that no matter what programmes we've put in place or how much money we've raised, it's simply not enough. And it isn't. In 1992, some 1.5 million people had HIV/AIDS. Today, it's 34 million. If that isn't an absolute emergency, I don't know what is.

Another thing that hasn't changed is the way we do business. The lessons we learned in those early days are important still; they remain the basis of our work and the key to our success. We still operate with a stream-lined staff of only three people in New York and nine in London. We still leverage partnerships in order to have as big an impact as possible. And our fidelity to

Over the years, the *Washington Post* has published a series of exposés detailing the failures of the city's Administration for HIV Policy and Programs. The stories they uncovered tie my stomach in knots. A city worker discovered boxes with thousands of records of people with AIDS that had never been entered into databases that the CDC and community-based organisations rely on to fight the disease.[2] Washington's underfunded AIDS surveillance team went for years without critical staff members, and thus couldn't even tell how bad the epidemic was in order to plan an appropriate response.[3] According to the *Post*, the city health department awarded $25 million 'to nonprofit agencies marked by questionable spending, a lack of clients, or lapses in record-keeping and care.'[4] Meanwhile, so many wonderful and deserving nonprofit groups that provide essential services in Washington are underfunded and short-staffed. I know this personally, because EJAF supports many amazing community organisations in the District of Columbia.

I could go on listing instances of despicable neglect when it comes to the AIDS epidemic in Washington. The more important point, however, is that countless people have died as a result.

The *Post* told the shocking story of one such victim, a fifty-year-old woman named Renee Paige. Renee had once been a vibrant presence in her neighbourhood, but she became terribly sick from AIDS. She was thrust into extreme poverty and, eventually, homelessness. After spending a freezing night on a park bench, unprotected from the pouring rain, Renee went to a community meeting, told her story, and begged for help. But none came. The *Post* reported that she died soon after, 'alone, on the bench, one mile from the HIV/AIDS Administration and within two miles of a dozen nonprofit groups that help people with AIDS.'[5]

How can this be? How can the capital of the United States of America have one of the most severe AIDS epidemics in the world? How can a woman with AIDS, like Renee, die practically around the corner from the bloody White House? It doesn't make any sense.

And yet, when you come to understand the nature of the AIDS epidemic, it makes *perfect* sense. The truth is as sad as it is simple. People like Renee will continue to die, and this epidemic will continue to spread, until we treat everybody suffering from HIV/AIDS with the very same level of dignity and compassion, no matter who they are or where they live.

Nowhere is this more apparent than in the United States, a country whose AIDS epidemic tells us so much about the AIDS epidemic everywhere. AIDS in America is not anywhere near the national emergency it is in countries such as South Africa, which has the highest number of people living with HIV/AIDS in the world. But the AIDS epidemic in the United States is serious. Roughly 1.2 million Americans are HIV-positive, and the CDC estimates 50,000 new infections each year. The rate of new infections has been steady at this level for several years, though the number of people who die of AIDS in America has greatly declined since 1995.

With that in mind, we should consider the following statistics:

As in Washington, DC, the majority of HIV-positive people in America are black, or gay, or both. African Americans make up only 14 per cent of the U.S. population, yet they represent 44 per cent of new infections. In 2009, black Americans had HIV infection rates seven times higher than whites. More to the point, AIDS was the third leading cause of death for middle-aged African American men and women in 2008. Rates of infection have sky-rocketed among gay men, especially among young gay and bisexual men who are black. In fact, 60 per cent of new infections are among gay or bisexual men overall. According to one CDC study involving twenty-one major U.S. cities, one in five gay men is HIV-positive.[6] Another study estimated that some 16.9 per cent of HIV-positive Americans spent time in federal or state correctional systems in 2006.[7] And 9 per cent of new infections are among injection drug users.

Let me be perfectly blunt, and unapologetically so: if we demonstrated the same compassion for gay men, poor people, minorities, sex workers, prisoners, and drug users that we do for other, less marginalised people, there would be no more AIDS in America. The reality is that until we give everybody the same access to treatment and prevention, AIDS will never, ever go away. It's that simple.

I don't mean to pick on America here. I adore and admire the United States. I'm a British citizen, of course, but I fell in love with America when I first visited back in 1970. I've lived part-time there for twenty years, and I spend much of the year in Atlanta and Los Angeles when I'm not on tour. America has given me a great deal, and it's my home as much as anywhere else in the world. And I should emphasise that America has done far more than any other nation to fight the AIDS epidemic. We would be absolutely nowhere without the life-saving research and actions taken by the U.S. government, the medical research community, and ultimately the American taxpayers.

However, my point is this:

AIDS, like every contagion, has evolved to take advantage of human weakness. A retrovirus, HIV is able to infiltrate our DNA, and it sabotages our immune system to the point that even ordinary infections become deadly. But what makes AIDS so frightening, so very lethal, is that it takes advantage of more than our biological weaknesses. It takes advantage of our *social* weaknesses. Indeed, what is truly killing tens of thousands of people in America and millions of people around the world is not just a virulent contagion but a lack of human compassion – a lack of love – for those who are living with HIV/AIDS.

AIDS might as well stand for 'Appalling Indifference to the Disenfranchised in Society.' The disease thrives, more than anything else, on our prejudice against those who are HIV-positive and most at risk of becoming infected. It thrives on bigotry and indifference toward the most vulnerable. Today, the 'deficiency' that kills almost 2 million people each year is not a microscopic virus called HIV; it is a macroscopic force called stigma. The 'syndrome' that has allowed AIDS to evolve into a global plague is not immunological; it is, quite simply, an absence of empathy for our fellow human beings.

It's a difficult thing to comprehend, but even if there *were* a cure for AIDS, it would not end the epidemic. Even if there *were* a vaccine to prevent HIV infection, inoculation alone would not stop the spread of the disease. This is not a pessimistic assessment; it is a realistic one, based on what is happening right now in the world.

We already have the tools and tactics that have been proven by research and science to halt the spread of the virus: condoms, health education, and needle exchange programmes. Yet conservative religious and political leaders continue to stand in the way of implementing what we know for a hard fact will save millions upon millions of lives.

We already have advanced treatments that not only allow those with HIV to live long and healthy lives but also prevent the spread of the disease – a miraculous discovery announced in 2011. Yet, right now, millions of people around the world – including in the richest nations – are at risk of dying in the near term, and transmitting the virus to their partners, because they don't have access to these life-saving medicines.

Of course, we must continue our search for a vaccine. We must pursue new research. But we must also summon the compassion needed to build a more equitable and just world.

The story of AIDS in Washington demonstrates what happens when we do not show compassion to those living with HIV/AIDS. But let me tell you another story, a story about the difference we can make when compassion drives our response to the AIDS epidemic.

In 1981, a woman named Elizabeth Glaser was nine months pregnant with her first child when she went into labour and began to hemorrhage badly. She lost so much blood that she had to be given multiple transfusions. Thankfully, her baby was delivered safely – a beautiful little girl whom Elizabeth and her husband, Paul, named Ariel.

Elizabeth, Paul, and Ariel were no ordinary family. Paul Michael Glaser was a famous actor, screenwriter, and director. At the time Ariel was born, he was known to millions as 'Starsky,' a star of the immensely popular 1970s television show *Starsky and Hutch*. Elizabeth, an accomplished woman in her own right, was a director at the Los Angeles Children's Museum. They were what you might call a power couple: well connected and well-to-do. Despite Elizabeth's life-threatening delivery, with the birth of Ariel, the Glasers had everything in the world going for them, and then some.

In 1985, when Ariel was four years old, she became very sick, and the doctors couldn't understand why. As a precaution, she was tested for HIV and, to the horror of her parents, was positive. The Glasers learned that Elizabeth had contracted HIV during the blood transfusion she received. Elizabeth had passed the virus to her daughter while breast-feeding. Paul and Elizabeth had since had a baby boy, Jake; he had the virus as well, having contracted it from Elizabeth while in her womb.

The entire family, except for Paul, was HIV-positive.

Facing the toxic stigma that surrounded AIDS at the time, Elizabeth and Paul withdrew Ariel from nursery school. They withdrew socially as well. Despite their fame and status within Hollywood, the Glasers were forced to suffer privately with those closest to them, while their doctors did the best they could to care for what was then an entirely untreatable disease.

In 1987, however, the FDA had approved the first AIDS treatment, AZT, which was demonstrated to delay, if only by a short while, the onset of full-blown AIDS in those with HIV. But Elizabeth and Paul quickly discovered that the government had not approved AZT for use in children like Ariel and Jake. The reason, they learned, was that paediatric AIDS had barely registered on the radar of the medical community, pharmaceutical companies, and policy makers. At the time, there were roughly a thousand cases of paediatric AIDS, and they represented only 2 per cent of the epidemic in the United States.

The bottom line was that the medical community wasn't responding quickly enough, and Elizabeth and Paul's little girl was dying.

In 1988, Ariel succumbed to AIDS. She was seven

years old. Elizabeth was distraught not only at the death of her young daughter but also at the thought – the seeming certainty – of losing her baby boy, Jake, as well.

Ariel's death transformed Elizabeth. She became a woman on a mission, and her single-minded focus was to bring attention and resources to bear on behalf of all HIV-positive children, including her son. Before Ariel died, and then months after burying her first child, Elizabeth travelled to Washington to share her painful story with members of Congress. While Elizabeth and her family's HIV-positive status was still unknown to the public and the press, she bravely confided in policy makers on Capitol Hill and implored them to help.

It worked. Congress soon voted to increase funding for paediatric AIDS research by $5 million. Elizabeth had made a real difference. But she didn't stop there. Through a family connection, she arranged a meeting with President Ronald Reagan and First Lady Nancy Reagan to share her story. They were moved, but little came of her White House visit; the research dollars just weren't flowing fast enough or to the extent necessary. And so Elizabeth decided to take matters into her own hands. She started a paediatric AIDS foundation to raise the money herself. Elizabeth was soon directing millions of dollars from her foundation to critical research that would have a tremendous impact.

In the meantime, the *National Enquirer* had seized on the Glasers' story. The tabloid published the details of their family tragedy for all of America to read, and they even went so far as to print photographs of little Ariel's grave. Elizabeth was understandably furious. She was suddenly thrust into the national spotlight.

Yet, with extraordinary poise, Elizabeth used the media attention, unwanted as it had been, to raise awareness about AIDS and its impact on children and adults alike. Her public advocacy culminated in her impassioned speech at the Democratic National Convention in 1992. She delivered sharp words to a national audience about presidents Reagan and Bush, criticising them for talking about their concern for those with HIV/AIDS while doing far too little to actually fight the epidemic.

Thankfully, Elizabeth succeeded where those two presidents failed. In the early 1990s, due primarily to her lobbying, Congress dedicated tens of millions of dollars to paediatric AIDS research. Eventually, scientists discovered how to prevent the transmission of HIV from mother to child. By the mid-2000s, only around 100 children in the United States were born with HIV each year, down from a peak of some 900 cases in 1992.

Today, the battle against the epidemic of paediatric

AIDS in America, and in much of the West, has largely been won. Very few American children contract HIV in utero, and practically none die of the disease.

Elizabeth didn't live to see this victory come to pass; she died of AIDS in 1994. But her impact and legacy live on through the Elizabeth Glaser Pediatric AIDS Foundation, which, over the years, has had a profound global impact. Today, the foundation carries on with the help of Elizabeth's son, Jake, now a young man who leads a vibrant, healthy life. Indeed, her work helped save his life.

But this work is far from over. While paediatric AIDS has been almost entirely extinguished in the United States and other developed countries, there are 3.4 *million* children infected globally and more than 1,000 new paediatric infections *each day*. Elizabeth's tragedy continues to unfold for countless mothers and their children.

Today, the worldwide epidemic of paediatric AIDS is so much worse than Elizabeth could have ever imagined. And yet, thanks to her, we know exactly how to end it. Indeed, we know how to end the disease not only among children but among all people, all over the world: with relentless compassion.

At the Democratic convention in 1992 – which she described as the most important week of her life

– Elizabeth told an audience of thousands at Madison Square Garden, and millions watching on television, how her AIDS-stricken daughter, Ariel, was the inspiration for her work:

> She taught me to love, when all I wanted to do was hate. She taught me to help others, when all I wanted to do was help myself. She taught me to be brave, when all I felt was fear.[8]

In her speech, Elizabeth called AIDS a 'crisis of caring.' She said that she was motivated not only by her own personal suffering, not only by her compassion for children, but also by her empathy for gay people, poor people, people of colour, and all who lived with the disease, and died from it, around the world.

Elizabeth's story shows us the way forward. It also begs the question, if we can end AIDS for children in America, why can't we end AIDS for everyone, everywhere?

The answer is that we *can* end AIDS. We simply haven't. Not yet.

6

Confronting Reality

South Africa is one of my very favourite places to visit. It's a magical country, and the people of that nation, having suffered through terrible hardship, are extraordinarily resilient. I have great love for them. I wish they had greater love for one another.

South Africa has one of the worst AIDS epidemics in the world, spread mainly by heterosexual sex. It also has one of the worst rape crises anywhere. This is no coincidence. The two are intertwined. By itself, rape is horrific. But for many women who are raped, the nightmare has just begun. According to one study, the rate of HIV infection is so high in South Africa that if a woman is raped by a man between twenty-five and forty-five years of age, there is at least a one-in-four chance that he is HIV-positive.[1]

In South Africa, a woman is raped every twenty-six seconds. But women aren't the only victims. Women and men, girls and boys, and horrifically even babies are victims of sexual assault. As the father of a young child, I have trouble contemplating such a thing. But it is terribly real, thanks in part to a poisonous superstition that having sex with a virgin is a cure for HIV/AIDS. Rape is so widespread in South Africa that some believe very young children and babies are the only sure virgins.

The situation is now out of control. In 2009, South Africa's Medical Research Council conducted a study surveying the extent of the rape crisis. Researchers found that one-quarter of the men interviewed admitted to raping someone.[2] Another study found that more than 60 per cent of boys over the age of eleven believed that 'sex is a male's natural entitlement and forcing a girl to have sex does not constitute a rape nor an act of violence.'[3]

If a society doesn't think there's anything wrong with rape, then anybody who speaks out against it will be stigmatised. One rape survivor in South Africa told the international relief organisation Médecins Sans Frontières, 'People laugh at me and say, "Oh, you will get HIV/AIDS now." These are my neighbours and people who live around me. They don't seem to think the men that raped me did anything wrong.'[4] When then vice president Jacob Zuma was on trial for rape, a charge of which he was acquitted, his supporters rallied to his cause, lobbing insults at his accuser and shouting, 'Burn the bitch,' outside the courthouse.[5]

In cases where rape victims are stigmatised, there are horrific consequences for the AIDS epidemic. Rapes are massively under-reported in South Africa, because of the shame associated with such violence and with being HIV-positive. Women who are raped fear they will be blamed or ostracised if they seek help or report the crime – they are shamed out of coming forward.

These fears are very well founded. Even if a woman goes to the authorities, it's unlikely she will get the help she needs. Rape survivors might wait by the roadside until police collect them, take them to the station to make a statement, and, many hours later, transport them to a hospital for examination and treatment. Police often dismiss these statements entirely. This highly demeaning and ineffective process seldom results in arrests of the perpetrators or help for rape survivors. So most women who are sexually assaulted face it alone. They wipe their own tears and find a way to move on.

But if rape survivors don't come forward, if they don't seek medical attention, they can't get access to emergency post-exposure prophylaxis (PEP) medicine, a type of anti-retroviral treatment that can prevent HIV infection within a short time after exposure. Thus, the rape and AIDS epidemics intertwine to form a vicious downward spiral.

My foundation decided to do something about the stigma surrounding rape and AIDS in South Africa, and the lack of care available for women and children who are sexually assaulted. Our intent was to offer the highest quality services to those for whom so little existed. To that end, in 2002 we joined with Médecins Sans Frontières and a network of more than fifteen local organisations to establish a twenty-four-hour, seven-day-a-week acute care centre that provides services to survivors of rape in Khayelitsha, a large township outside Cape Town. The centre, called Simelela, is the first of its kind in South Africa. In Xhosa, the local language, 'Simelela' means 'to lean on.'

Simelela provides medical services, and it also tries to combat the stigma of rape and violence against women by empowering them to gain more control over their sexual lives. Women can walk in off the street, day or night, and receive treatment. Workers at the clinic bring women in need of help to the centre. Shockingly, girls under the age of fourteen make up one-third of Simelela's clients. But the good news is that Simelela can help them. Staff members give all clients post-rape medical care, PEP treatment to prevent HIV for those who need it, and a forensic examination, and they work with clients to make a detailed police report as well. Women and children who visit Simelela are treated with dignity, care, and love.

Before Simelela, this level of support for rape victims was sadly lacking. But today, thanks to the dedication and hard work of the centre's caregivers, Cape Town's rape and HIV epidemics are being tackled head-on, and with real results. Not a single client of the centre who has been given PEP treatment has contracted HIV. And, not long after Simelela was founded, the clinic was seeing more rape clients in a month than the only previous available service – some fifteen kilometres away – saw in a year. Today, the staff at Simelela also work with local police, other clinics, and courts to ensure that every woman's confidentiality is protected and that she is supported every step of the way.

Simelela has grown and started to extend its reach. It is now recognised as a model of post-rape care for South Africa. Indeed, Simelela's model is even being incorporated at a new district hospital in the middle of Khayelitsha to provide a flagship service for women and children who have been raped.

We still have a very long way to go. Changing people's attitudes about women, about HIV, and about sexual violence won't happen overnight. But the very fact that rape survivors in Khayelitsha now have a place to seek help is a tremendous victory. Building a rape crisis centre, acknowledging that rape is in fact a crisis and that survivors need services – these are monumental steps. Simelela is beginning to break the stigma surrounding sexual violence.

When I visited the Simelela centre in 2007, I met an extraordinary young woman named Fumana. She was raped by her cousin when she was only eight years old. She didn't tell anyone. Later she tested positive for HIV. But she told me the most remarkable thing. Today she says that she is *proud* to know her HIV status. She is proud because most people are afraid to talk about the disease, afraid to talk about rape, so they don't get tested, they don't know their status. But this beautiful, healthy woman knows about her disease, she is getting treatment for it, and she is *empowered* as a survivor of sexual violence. Fumana speaks out about what she endured, and in doing so she is helping to break the stigma surrounding the disease. In fact, Fumana is now studying forensics, so she too can support victims of rape.

I was deeply moved to meet her. I told her that in sharing her story and in talking about her status, she is a real hero. The more voices that are heard, the more heroes who come forward, the less society can ignore the reality of rape and AIDS in South Africa. I should note that Fumana's story and EJAF's work with Simelela have inspired our support of services at clinics in Uganda and Kenya, serving thousands of women. Fumana, through her bravery, has helped them all.

I'm very proud of the work that Simelela does. I know it makes a difference. But how many South African women have been raped since you started reading this chapter? How many children have had their innocence torn from them? How many people will be infected with HIV because stigma keeps them from getting the education, the services, and the treatment they need to prevent it? How many will die as a result?

AIDS will never end until we confront the reality of the epidemic and how it spreads. That means directly addressing the most difficult issues facing society, including poverty, drug use, sexual identity, and, yes, sexual violence. And the only way to do that, the only way to face these truths, is to overcome our own prejudices, to overcome stigma.

It is stigma that keeps us from doing what is necessary to end this epidemic. It is stigma that keeps us from confronting reality. To end AIDS, we must end stigma. It's the single biggest obstacle to stopping the global epidemic. I've seen how people's lives can be ruined because of it. I've seen how society's response to the AIDS epidemic can be warped by it. But I've also seen how, with time and effort, stigma can be alleviated.

John Scott once told me about how, in 1993, he and our very close friend Eli Saleeby, one of the founding board members of EJAF, went to visit a friend of theirs who was suffering from full-blown AIDS. When John and Eli arrived at their friend's apartment in Atlanta, he was so sick that he had to be taken to the hospital right away. Their friend was transported in a special ambulance for AIDS patients, because, as I said, during the early years of the epidemic, even health-care workers were needlessly frightened of people with HIV/AIDS.

The ambulance took John and Eli's friend to an indigent care facility in downtown Atlanta, but John and Eli wanted to make sure he received the best medical treatment possible, so they arranged for their friend to be moved to Grady Hospital, the city's major medical centre. At this point, John and Eli's friend was incredibly sick with vomiting and diarrhoea, and he was in terrible pain. But once he arrived at Grady Hospital, he sat on a gurney in a hallway for almost twenty-four hours. For an entire day, he just lay there, wasting away in his own suffering, his own humiliation, like he didn't matter at all. No one wanted to deal with him, to be near him, to treat him. Such was the stigma surrounding AIDS in a major American hospital in 1993.

Fast-forward to 2010, when Eli himself had been living with HIV for nineteen years. Eventually, he developed severe complications, including lymphoma. It happened so quickly that by the time Eli's doctors began treating the cancer it had already spread like wildfire. John got a call one day. Eli had fallen in a pharmacy parking lot and didn't know who or where he was. John got on the first flight he could and arrived at the exact same hospital he and Eli had taken their friend to nearly twenty years earlier, Grady Hospital in Atlanta. John couldn't help but think of the experience they'd had there before.

But this time, it was a completely different story. John didn't find Eli abandoned as an untouchable in some hallway. To the contrary, Eli had a six-person medical team. They immediately briefed John. They walked him through his friend's condition. They treated Eli, and John for that matter, with total respect and compassion. They didn't care about Eli's disease – they cared about Eli. And they did everything they could for him. Sadly, Eli passed away, but he did so in peace and with the dignity that he deserved.

Fighting stigma is difficult work. Over time, it can – and will – be overcome, but only when we acknowledge what stigma is, how it works, and why it is so deadly when it comes to HIV/AIDS. There has been plenty of research done on stigma, studies conducted and published by people far more knowledgeable than myself. I'm no expert, but anyone can understand the basics. We've all seen it and experienced it.

Consider how we often stigmatise the way people look – someone's height, weight, or a physical feature or deformity that strays from what we think is 'normal.' Another kind of stigma is rooted in moral or religious judgements. We impose our own values on others, and condemn them for falling outside what we think is the 'right' way to live. We see addicts as 'weak-willed,' for example, or homosexuals as 'sinful', and we marginalise them accordingly. And then there's the age-old stigma based on various differences among people – for instance, their race, class, faith, gender, ethnicity, nationality, or sexual identity.[6]

AIDS touches on many of these stigmas at once. The illness can be visible and debilitating. It's spread through sex and shared needles. It disproportionately impacts gays, minorities, and the poor. Very quickly, we've built up several layers of stigma. The more layers there are, the more difficult they are to peel back and to remove.[7]

This is the heart of the AIDS crisis and why it is so very difficult to beat. Thanks to stigma, instead of directing our animosity and fear at someone's disease, we direct it at the person who is sick. Ultimately, this makes the epidemic even worse. HIV-positive people are pushed into the shadows. They often do not receive treatment or care, because they are afraid to make public their HIV status. They are afraid to tell their families and their doctors. They are afraid to seek treatment. They are ashamed. And this shame is deadly.

Recently, someone I've known for a very long time confided in me that he had tested HIV-positive. He was so scared to tell me that he could hardly look me in the eye. He thought that I would be angry with him, that I would reject him. He thought that I would tell him he'd been irresponsible and that I would no longer want to be his friend. He said, 'Elton, will you forgive me?' I was stunned. I replied, 'What do you mean, forgive you? There's nothing to forgive. You haven't done anything wrong. You're my friend and I love you.' Here he was, feeling scared about the disease, ashamed to tell an old friend, and upset with himself for contracting HIV all at once. This is the danger of stigma. You can't overestimate what a powerful force it is.

And it's a very old force, at that. AIDS is not the first disease to be stigmatised, of course. Not by a long shot. Venereal diseases such as syphilis, for example, have long been stigmatised as an indication of a person's sexual and moral life. Throughout history, people with syphilis were shunned and scorned. In the United States, for instance, immigrant populations were singled out as particularly prone to the disease and likely to spread it. People who already hated immigrants had one more reason to loathe them.

Even non-venereal diseases have long been stigmatised. In 1832 a cholera epidemic broke out in New York neighbourhoods where poor, ethnic minorities and immigrants were concentrated. It was thought that the disease was spread by 'immoral' sexual behaviour and alcohol use. And the cramped, dirty, and unhygienic quarters in which these impoverished communities resided – and which certainly contributed to the spread of disease – became the subject of society's contempt, instead of its concern. Rich people thought of cholera as something that only impacted the poor. Thus, it went untreated. This lack of compassion, rooted in stigma, allowed cholera to eventually spread unchecked to the general population. Of course, it wasn't until the disease went mainstream that society started to do something about it.[8]

A century and a half later, the AIDS epidemic followed a similar course. It began in the 1980s as a 'gay disease.' At the time, homophobia kept the U.S. government from allowing funding for any educational programmes or materials that included instructions on how to have safe homosexual sex. Thanks to people such as Senator Jesse Helms, federal funding was banned for any AIDS education materials that seemed to support or encourage, even indirectly, 'homosexual activities.'[9] In other words, you couldn't teach gay men how to have safe sex. Of course, this allowed HIV to spread, and spread, and spread. Had the government cared about gay people, had homosexuals not been so stigmatised, the epidemic could have been, to some extent, contained. But the government didn't care about gays, HIV spread uncontrollably, and we are suffering the impact of that indifference to this day.

Sadly, governments haven't yet learned the fundamental lesson that to beat an infectious disease you must treat everyone equally, with compassion, and with dignity. I was reminded of this while on the European leg of my concert tour in 2010. Reading the paper over breakfast one morning, I came across a horrible story. In Malawi, Tiwonge Chimbalanga, a transgender woman, and Steven Monjeza, a man, had each been sentenced to fourteen years of hard labour in prison. They had been prosecuted for committing 'indecent acts.' Their crime had been nothing more than being in love.

I was stunned and disgusted. Malawi has a terrible AIDS epidemic, one of the worst anywhere. Almost 12 per cent of the population between the ages of fifteen and forty-nine is HIV-positive. More than 50,000 people die of AIDS each year. That's why EJAF has worked in Malawi since 1998, assisting with treatment and prevention efforts. In 2006, we co-funded an effort by Médecins Sans Frontières in the district of Thyolo to help the government provide universal access to treatment for all HIV-positive Malawians. It has been a great success, in no small part because of the government's own policy of non-discrimination when it comes to access to care. Everyone should theoretically be able to get treatment, including gays.

When I learned of the persecution and prosecution of Chimbalanga and Monjeza, my first thought was of the terrible injustice of their situation. I then thought of the destructive impact the government's actions would have on our HIV treatment and prevention work in Malawi. With the threat of prosecution looming, gay people would be far less likely to seek treatment through a government programme. By stigmatising a subgroup, by making a legal example of them, the Malawian government was driving AIDS further into the shadows, perpetuating the epidemic they were hoping to end. This sort of state-sanctioned discrimination costs lives, and it was counter to the work EJAF was funding in Malawi. I didn't keep these thoughts to myself, of course; I wrote an open letter to the Malawian president, Bingu wa Mutharika, that was published by *The Guardian*. Luckily, Chimbalanga and Monjeza were pardoned, and they were spared their unjust sentences.

Reading about Chimbalanga and Monjeza, I also couldn't help but think back to the day I was legally bound to the man I love. David and I had been together at that point for twelve years. It was important to both of us to obtain our civil partnership on the very first day it became legal in Britain: 21 December 2005. We went to the town hall in Windsor, and honestly we weren't sure what to expect. We thought some hateful people might react negatively to the idea of same-sex partnerships. We worried they might take out their bigotry on us. And we were happy, and very relieved, when we received nothing but warm wishes on that special day. Not one hateful or bigoted sentiment was expressed. And it's been that way ever since.

David and I are an openly gay couple, very much in love, very much in the public eye, and people treat us wonderfully everywhere in the world, from Africa to Asia to the Middle East. Of course, we aren't your ordinary gay couple. We are celebrities, and I know we're treated differently because of it. And yet, the acceptance David and I are very fortunate to experience makes me hopeful that, one day, gay people everywhere will be embraced for who they are and treated just the same as we are treated, and just the same as straight couples are treated. All people, including Chimbalanga and Monjeza, should be allowed to love each other openly and in peace the way David and I do. Unfortunately, the vast majority of gay people around the world suffer some degree of homophobia. In fact, homosexuality is banned in too many places to name. Gay sex is a crime in more than seventy-six countries.[10]

Discrimination against gays is wrong, but it's so much more than that. Homophobia harms everyone in the societies in which it is prevalent, because it hinders health education, it frustrates activities that could help prevent the spread of HIV, and it discourages people from seeking treatment. In Uganda, for instance, a radio station was fined when one of its programmes discussed the need for HIV/AIDS services for gay men.[11] In India, people have been arrested, beaten, and charged under anti-sodomy laws for giving out information on safe sex.[12] Gay people in many African countries are at greater risk of contracting the disease because they are less likely to receive information and treatment.

Fighting homophobia is central to fighting AIDS, because the stigma associated with being gay prevents the response we need to beat the disease.

To understand this, consider the AIDS epidemic in Thailand, as detailed in a recent report by amfAR.[13]

Many Asian countries, including Thailand, have been waging war against AIDS for decades, and some have made some real progress. But almost all of them have failed to make a dent in the spread of AIDS among gay men because homosexuality in many Asian communities is terribly stigmatised. This has certainly been the case in Thailand.

In the mid-'80s, Thailand's Ministry of Public Health knew of only forty-three reported AIDS cases. There were almost no prevention efforts in place, as the government didn't think of AIDS as a real problem. In 1987, the official rate of AIDS was almost zero. But by 1989, it had risen to between 18 and 52 per cent among different groups of injection drug users. In just one year, from June 1988 to late 1989, the rate went from zero to 43 per cent among female sex workers in Chiang Mai.

Naturally, the government took notice. They smartly instituted a range of prevention efforts, including a condom campaign that was estimated to prevent 8 million new infections. They were aggressive and successful. Rates of extramarital sex went down. Brothel visits decreased. Condom use increased. The results were meaningful and led to a dramatic decline in new HIV infections, from 143,000 new infections in 1991 to 19,000 in 2003. In 2004, the global AIDS community convened in Bangkok at the XV International AIDS Conference, in part to mark Thailand's successful response and tout it as an example to be replicated elsewhere.

But here's the problem: the government's anti-AIDS campaigns never targeted men who have sex with men. That was too uncomfortable, too taboo. And so this community in Thailand was ignored. It's no surprise, then, that things kept getting worse. Men continued to have unprotected sex with each other. They continued to contract HIV at alarming rates. They continued to die. While HIV infection rates among other groups in Thailand were going down, the infection rate for men who had sex with men in Bangkok was sky-rocketing. In 2003, it was over 17 per cent. By 2005, 28 per cent were HIV-positive.

To me, Thailand is a perfect example of what's wrong with today's AIDS response. It's a perfect example of how stigma spreads AIDS. The government of Thailand saw a problem. They saw their people getting sick and dying. To their great credit, they reached out to marginalised populations and the general public alike. They provided critical prevention information and programmes to drug users, prostitutes, and the poor. It's amazing, really, how much of an effort the government made to reach traditionally stigmatised populations.

But the stigma against homosexuality ran so deep that it could not be overcome. And for that reason, among others, Thailand still has a very serious AIDS epidemic on its hands.

When it comes to homophobia, what's true in the developing world is true of Western countries as well. According to the CDC, the only group in the United States with HIV rates that significantly increased between 2006 and 2009 were gay and bisexual men, and particularly black gay and bisexual men under the age of thirty.[14] And it's no surprise. Homosexuality is still incredibly stigmatised in America, and particularly in the African American community.

There are so many stigmas to confront, so many that must be peeled back to expose the reality of the AIDS epidemic. Many of them relate to sex or sexual identity. After all, sex is how HIV is most commonly spread. But it's also spread through injection drug use, which is responsible for some 9 per cent of new HIV infections in the United States. Sharing needles is common among addicts. Needles cost money, after all, and when you're hooked on heroin, your only thought is being able to afford the drug itself. Why buy a needle when you can borrow one? Tragically, this is how so many people have contracted HIV, by sharing a needle with someone who has the virus.

Fortunately, there's a very easy way to prevent the spread of HIV among those who use injection drugs. Needle exchange programmes provide clean needles to active drug users. It's a straightforward and inexpensive means of preventing new cases of HIV. It's also effective in fighting addiction, because most needle exchange programmes serve as a bridge for people to enter drug treatment. That's exactly what we need to get people off drugs and to curb the spread of HIV all at once. The world's first needle exchange programme was set up as early as 1984 in Amsterdam. Thanks to a robust effort of needle exchange and widespread HIV testing, counselling, and drug treatment programmes in Amsterdam, over time there have been significant reductions not only in HIV but also in diseases such as hepatitis B.[15] Needle exchange programmes have had amazing success in that city and many others.

Needle exchange clearly works. But in the United States, it's against the law for the federal government to spend money on needle exchange programmes. And there is only one reason for such a ridiculous policy: stigma.

Many American politicians are opposed to such programmes on moral or political grounds. They don't like the idea of using tax dollars for a service that helps rather than punishes drug users, even if doing so prevents the spread of a deadly disease and helps transition active users off drugs. Conservative members of Congress have successfully blocked federal funding for needle exchange programmes for two decades, despite the fact that studies by government health agencies, including the National Institutes of Health, have found that these programmes really work.[16] In 2009, Congress finally voted to allow federal support for needle exchange. Unfortunately, in 2012, Congress reinstated its ban for political reasons.

A national, federally funded needle exchange programme in America could prevent 4,000 new HIV infections per year. It could drastically reduce the incidence of AIDS. It could also drastically curb drug use. For heaven's sake, it could even save money spent on law enforcement, hospitalisation for the uninsured, and treatment programmes for those living with HIV. It would pay for itself. But thanks to the stigma surrounding drug use, the U.S. government willfully ignores the health and well-being of vulnerable addicts. It ignores the reality of drugs and AIDS in America. This costs lives in a very real, and very tragic, way.

Even in America, even after thirty years of the AIDS epidemic, even after the tremendous progress we've made in understanding and treating HIV/AIDS, the stigma surrounding the disease is significant. Today, thirty-four

American states have criminal laws that punish HIV-positive people for exposing another person to the virus – even if there's no actual risk, no actual transmission. Too many HIV-positive people are now in prison, serving absurdly long sentences, for alleged 'crimes' such as biting and spitting. It doesn't matter that there's no way to transmit HIV through saliva. The stigma is so bad that it has warped the nation's laws and ruined countless lives.

In 2011, I saw an incredible short film, 'HIV Is Not a Crime,' which was produced and directed by Sean Strub, a longtime AIDS activist and a real hero of the movement. It tells heartbreaking stories of Americans whose lives have been destroyed thanks to legal prosecution based on their HIV status.[17]

Nick Rhoades, for example, had an undetectable viral load, used a condom, and did not transmit HIV to his partner. However, he and his partner later broke up, they became estranged, and his ex-partner pressed charges against Nick on grounds of his HIV status alone. Nick was charged with a class B felony, which is on par with manslaughter and kidnapping. He was convicted, sentenced to twenty-five years in prison, and deemed a lifetime sex offender. Of his trial and sentencing, Nick said, 'HIV. Gay. Sex. It's like a gift, wrapped up on a platter [for prosecutors]. It doesn't matter what the facts are or the science.'

Ultimately, Nick was spared the twenty-five-year sentence and instead put on five years of probation. He had to register as a sex offender every three months, he couldn't visit social networking websites, and he had to wear a GPS ankle bracelet to be monitored twenty-four hours a day. For being HIV-positive, he was treated like a fully fledged criminal.

Sean's film also tells the story of a woman, Monique, who had been prosecuted under a similar law. While she insisted on safe sex, she hadn't disclosed her HIV status to her partner. Monique was afraid of the stigma surrounding HIV in her community. She was later prosecuted for not telling her partner that she was HIV-positive. Monique's prosecution only validated her worst fears about how society would respond to her disease.

The stigma surrounding AIDS creates a vicious and deadly cycle. It encourages those with HIV to hide their status because they are afraid of being not only ostracised but also criminalised. It encourages society to blame those with HIV. It rationalises pre-existing prejudices. It stymies the response we need to curb the epidemic. Indeed, it causes the epidemic to spread. In fact, stigma is a major reason why the epidemic is worsening among certain populations, even while we're making progress among others.

Is it any wonder there is a high incidence of AIDS among injection drug users in countries where injection drug use is stigmatised? Is it any wonder rape is a major cause of HIV transmission in South Africa, where rape itself is a cause of shame for women and a reality that society long refused to acknowledge, let alone confront?

In one article I read, the head of the Northeast Florida AIDS Network in Jacksonville said that she had trouble finding office space for the organisation. Landlords refused to rent to them because they didn't want people with AIDS in their buildings.[18] Is it any wonder, then, that Jacksonville, Florida, has the third highest rate of new AIDS cases among American cities? Is it any wonder that some 240,000 Americans have HIV but don't know it, when HIV has been criminalised in the majority of American states? Who would want to know their HIV status when testing positive could land them behind bars?

In a twisted way, it all makes sense. The places where stigma is the worst have the worst AIDS epidemics. That's because stigma itself prevents an appropriate response to the disease. It not only perpetuates the epidemic; stigma makes the epidemic impossible to beat.

But here's the thing: If the entire world, every government, every charity, every individual, decided tomorrow that needle exchange wasn't a bad thing, that we should, in fact, start needle exchange programmes all over the world, programmes that would reach every last injection drug user, we would eliminate the disease from that population. And yet AIDS would still exist in Uganda, where homosexuality is illegal and punishable by death. AIDS would still exist in Bangladesh, where female sex workers are denied their rights, are frequently victims of violence, and are almost totally unable to protect themselves from the disease because they are stigmatised. AIDS would still exist in South Africa, where HIV is spread largely through heterosexual sex and where the stigma around sexual violence complicates society's response.

Unless we eradicate stigma everywhere, we will never eradicate AIDS everywhere.

7

The Heart of the Matter

I'm far from the first person to preach the importance of compassion, indeed the *need* for compassion, when it comes to combating AIDS. Long before I ever got into this work, many brilliant, dedicated professionals from all around the world were orchestrating a compassionate response to the epidemic. I'm simply, and humbly, following in their footsteps. And while I would never suggest that I'm an AIDS expert, I have seen quite a lot through the work of my foundation.

Over the years, I've had the opportunity to meet some of the greatest heroes in the global fight against AIDS. They include my many extraordinary colleagues around the world who are in the trenches, day after day. I've been lucky enough to travel the world and visit dozens of projects that EJAF has funded. I've seen the difference these heroes are making. Compassion is a nice sentiment, but it's so much more than that. I've seen with my own eyes what's possible when compassion is put into practice. The organisations that my foundation supports have made incredible progress in fighting stigma and AIDS through their compassionate policies and programmes.

I try to spread this message everywhere I go, and it's not always well received. In 2007, my foundation organised a free concert in Ukraine to raise awareness about the terrible AIDS crisis in that country. Sadly, religious groups encouraged people to boycott us. They believed that gay people were responsible for the spread of AIDS and that I was promoting homosexual propaganda. Nevertheless, on the day of the concert, from behind my piano that June evening, I was stunned and overjoyed to see hundreds of thousands of people, including many religious leaders, packed into Independence Square in Kiev. They were undeterred by the bigotry and the stigma surrounding homosexuality and AIDS. I told the crowd that I was there to support their country's fight against HIV/AIDS, and I asked them to find the courage to show love and support to all those living with the disease. The crowd roared, and it filled me with hope. It made me think of how far we'd come since EJAF had first started working in Ukraine, five years earlier, in 2002.

Ukraine has the worst epidemic of HIV/AIDS in Eastern Europe, with more than 400,000 people infected and the fastest-growing rate of new infections in the world. The epidemic there is a classic example of how stigma and fear work hand in hand with the disease, spreading it further, killing people faster.

Sixty per cent of infected Ukrainians are tragically young, between the ages of twenty and thirty-four. At the greatest risk are 100,000 homeless young people in major cities such as Kiev, Odessa, and Donetsk. You'll find them sprawled on crumbling streets or in abandoned buildings, relics of the Soviet era. Many of them turn to prostitution to survive; 35 per cent of those who do have HIV/AIDS. Others numb their painful lives by injecting cheaply concocted drugs, like a cocktail called 'screw' made of surgical liquid, cough syrup, and the phosphorous tips of matches. More than 40 per cent of these drug-addicted, homeless youths are HIV-positive.[1]

These young people, and many other HIV-positive Ukrainians around the country, have often been treated with contempt by religious groups, by their communities, by people who think AIDS is brought on by sin. They are shunned. Spat upon. Ostracised. Made to feel worthless. Having your humanity wholly rejected because of whatever you're going through is the worst thing that can happen to you. As I've said, not to be cared for or cared about, not to even be thought about, is the most painful feeling a human being can ever experience. To make people feel as though they are completely on their own in their struggles, that they are invisible to everybody else, regardless of their circumstances, is utterly inhumane. For far too long, this was exactly the plight of those who were sick and dying of AIDS in Ukraine.

The Ukrainian government was not entirely indifferent to the problem. In 2000, the authorities paid it appropriate lip service, calling the situation a national emergency. But what happened next, unfortunately, is what happens in many other countries. The government developed an unsound, incoherent, and underfunded policy framework to combat the disease. It was a plan in name only. They made fancy-sounding decrees, passed a few laws, created a few programmes. But on the ground, in the lives of real people – especially stigmatised people – nothing happened. Nothing changed.

In the meantime, the disease spread. Prostitutes, drug users, gay people, young people, all of whom had the highest rates of the disease, were afraid to seek treatment. Who would, in the face of such bigotry? Gay men in particular were terrified of what would happen if they came out of the shadows. Those who did were basically told, 'There's nothing we can do for you. Go home and die.'

When EJAF first started working in Ukraine, there were only a few clinics where people could safely get the care they needed. One such safe haven was the Lavra Clinic in Kiev, right next door to the city's historic Orthodox church, the Kiev-Pechersk Lavra, or Monastery of the Caves. People with HIV/AIDS from all over Ukraine did whatever it took – walked, bused, hitchhiked, crawled, used all their savings – to make their way to Lavra for life-saving treatment in a supportive and non-discriminatory environment.

But to address such a large and fast-growing epidemic, much more mobilisation was needed. So EJAF got involved with an amazing group called the All Ukrainian Network of People Living with HIV/AIDS, or AUKN for short. It's an organisation of HIV-positive people, some of the most marginalised in Ukraine, a group of ex-drug users, the pariahs, the hopeless. We worked with them for about three years to help build their organisation and set up a variety of programmes throughout the country. Initially, AUKN was reaching around 1,700 people each month. Today, their impact has grown more than thirtyfold, connecting some 57,000 people living with HIV/AIDS and 5,500 children affected by the disease with the services they need. As a network of people infected and affected by HIV them-selves, they are also breaking down the stigma and discrimination that serve as barriers to treatment by reaching 53,000 prisoners with HIV testing.

AUKN embodies a critical tenet of EJAF's work. You have to go where the disease is. You have to look squarely at the darkest realities of our society and find those who are at the fringes, who are suffering the most. These are the people who need our help. And, as it turns out, these are also the people who can alter the course of the epidemic.

By 2007, AUKN was widely respected and hailed for its successful work. In fact, when the Ukrainian Ministry of Health was shown to be so corrupt that the Global Fund to Fight AIDS, Tuberculosis, and Malaria wouldn't finance its AIDS programmes, AUKN stepped in. The Global Fund selected AUKN as Ukraine's official recipient of a major grant to fight AIDS. This network of the dispossessed now manages the Global Fund's $51.9 million AIDS treatment and care budget for all of Ukraine! Of course, they were able to do this because, years earlier, EJAF saw them not only as people who deserve better but also as agents of change. Our compassion was empowering to them. And they became quite powerful, indeed. AUKN, working with a consortium of partners including the William J. Clinton Foundation, was able to successfully force the government to reform the notoriously corrupt drug procurement process in

Ukraine. As a result, the price of AIDS medicines dropped 90 per cent, doubling the number of people the government could afford to treat.

Working with AUKN and witnessing their incredible achievements encouraged us to get involved with other organisations in Ukraine. Today, we are also supporting training for child-care specialists to work with HIV-positive children across the country. And we're funding the establishment of six sites specifically to provide services for gay men, who will be able to get information, condoms, and referrals for testing and treatment. In a country that still deals with rampant homophobia, this is a huge breakthrough.

The head of AUKN and many of its founding members came to my 2007 concert in Kiev. It was the first chance I had to meet them in person. The founder of AUKN told Anne Aslett, the executive director of EJAF in the United Kingdom, and me, 'When no one else wanted to have anything to do with us, it was the Elton John AIDS Foundation that believed in us, that believed that our group played a central role in the solution to the problem.' Now, the Ukrainian govern-ment lauds their work. The international community acknowledges their achievements. They're making important progress on the ground.

That's the power of compassion. That's the virtuous

cycle we must replicate the world over in order to beat the AIDS epidemic.

One of the places most in need of such a virtuous cycle is Haiti, where extreme poverty and the stigma surrounding sexual identity complicate that country's vicious AIDS epidemic. One of EJAF's grantees in Haiti is an organisation called Fondation SEROvie. Since 1997, SEROvie has been the first and only institution in Haiti to provide health services to – and advocate for the rights of – lesbian, gay, bisexual, and transgender (LGBT) people. By focusing on both health care and human rights, SEROvie is trying to break the cycle of discrimination, poverty, and AIDS in a country with an extremely high HIV infection rate of 1.9 per cent.

My foundation first got involved with SEROvie in 2007, through our partnership with an amfAR initiative targeting men who have sex with men around the world. It's another example of our lessons learned at work: connect with reputable organisations that have enormous reach, like amfAR, and build partnerships on the ground with other groups, like SEROvie, that know exactly what people need and how resources should be spent.

In the Haitian capital, Port-au-Prince, SEROvie does everything from distributing condoms to sending peer educators to the homes of HIV-infected people. This is difficult work in an impoverished society with tremendous stigma against gay and transgender people. Many of SEROvie's clients are already very poor and therefore more likely to engage in risky, transactional sex to earn money. Through our partnership with amfAR, we supported SEROvie's vocational training programme to give young men the skills they need to support themselves in a healthy way instead. This was just one of the many amazing projects the organisation was running.

But everything changed at 4:53 p.m. on 12 January 2010, when a 7.0-magnitude earthquake reduced much of Port-au-Prince to rubble. SEROvie's executive director, Steeve Laguerre, has since described the horror of that moment: 'We were having our usual support group meeting on a quiet Tuesday afternoon when the worst happened. The sound is unforgettable. I can't even describe the horror as the ceiling and the wall of the conference room started to fall and the chaos started.'[2] That day, SEROvie lost fourteen of its staff members.

The earthquake exacerbated the already overwhelming AIDS crisis in Haiti. Many HIV/AIDS clinics were destroyed, many health workers were killed. Almost no one could get access to badly needed medication. It wasn't too long afterward that the executive director of EJAF in the United States, Scott Campbell, went to

Haiti to see first hand just how bad things were. What he witnessed was heart-breaking and deeply frustrating. But he also saw cause for hope. Since the earthquake flattened SEROvie's home, the staff was operating out of tents. They were relentless. No amount of tragedy or turmoil could keep them down. They had not given up.

At the same time, their work was harder than ever. When the infrastructure of the country was decimated, the LGBT community, which was already marginalised, became further isolated. They lost their support networks and safe spaces. As one lesbian in Port-au-Prince said, 'Loneliness, invisibility, and social isolation are persistent problems for us.'[3] SEROvie had always been a haven for these stigmatised populations, and now even that was gone. Family and friends who previously provided support and shelter were scattered. Try to imagine how terrifying it would be to live in a place where your only protection from violence and bigotry was the lock on the door of your home. Now try to imagine the fear when that home – with its door and its lock – came crashing down. When he visited, Scott said the fear was palpable.

The discrimination that the LGBT community faced after the earthquake is hard to stomach. Many gay men reported physical assault, rape, and even being denied aid. One young gay man named Lengemy told SEROvie that he was kicked out of an emergency food distribution line.[4] Can you imagine that, in the midst of one of the worst humanitarian crises ever experienced by a country, people were being denied the basic necessities for survival because of prejudice, because of sexual orientation?

Some of this, strangely enough, was a function of good intentions. As a matter of general disaster policy, food aid is distributed only to women because they are more likely to get it to family members. But many gay men don't have women in their families. When SEROvie sent a letter to the American Red Cross requesting an exception to that policy, the organisation was told to consult with the Haitian Red Cross, because they couldn't give targeted assistance to specific minority populations. Believing that the Haitian Red Cross wouldn't help, SEROvie didn't bother.[5]

Still, SEROvie kept serving the people who flocked to them. In the face of incredible challenges, not the least of which was being forced to operate out of tents, the organisation quickly reassembled and got to work. Steeve Laguerre says that the key to success is to listen to what people want and need – or, to put it another way, to demonstrate compassion to those who are suffering. Initially, SEROvie spent a lot of time and resources providing counselling and distributing what little rice, cornmeal, and cooking oil they had. Then they shifted their focus to other basic needs like shelter and safety. To prevent the spread of waterborne diseases brought on after the earthquake, they taught their clients about decontaminating water, keeping their living spaces clean, and using mosquito nets. They also continued their work to prevent the spread of HIV/AIDS. EJAF is now helping SEROvie to establish an HIV testing and counselling clinic in its Port-au-Prince office, the only clinic in Haiti that will address the specific needs of the LGBT community.

Like many of the successful programmes that EJAF partners with, SEROvie addresses its clients as whole people. They look at their needs and help them live their lives with self-respect and dignity. Whether that involves giving them the means to access affordable housing, the confidence and skills to find good work, or the discipline to take their medicine every day, SEROvie treats each individual as worthy of care. As a result, they are able to help address other aspects of people's lives that make them vulnerable to HIV/AIDS, as well as many other diseases.

Despite how much time has passed since the 2010 earthquake, life is still extremely challenging for LGBT Haitians, especially those living with HIV/AIDS. While he was in Port-au-Prince, Scott heard the most horrific stories. One man was reportedly raped by four other men – but when he went to the police to report the attack, they laughed at him. They said that since he was gay, he must have enjoyed it.

I can't imagine what it must be like to keep waking up every day to help another client with a dreadful situation. To fight another battle with the authorities. To do impossible work in impossible circumstances. But SEROvie keeps going – and they're making progress. They have stepped up their advocacy efforts and are training government officials, law enforcement, and others to reduce the stigma and discrimination their clients face. They are working relentlessly toward a society that protects, not persecutes, its citizens living with HIV/AIDS. They are trying to start a virtuous cycle, and EJAF will continue to help them do so.

We're also hoping to trigger such cycles in America. There, the AIDS epidemic is very different from Haiti's, but not as different as you might think. As it turns out, in developing and developed countries alike, the fight against AIDS comes down to compassion.

I love the American South, where I've spent much of my life. I am always blown away by how beautiful that part of the country is. There's something especially magical about Southwest Louisiana. Cypress trees that frame the haunting bayou. Flooded rice paddies and lonely prairies without a house or a living soul for miles. It's one of the most rural places in America. And as with much of rural America, there is a quiet but deadly AIDS crisis that has been simmering for decades. Nearly 1,000 people in this one small corner of Louisiana are HIV-positive. They are among the poorest, most marginalised people in the nation. And they are mostly African American.

The HIV/AIDS epidemic is raging in the African American community nationally, and especially in the South. As I've said, almost half of all HIV diagnoses are among African Americans. Shockingly, AIDS is a leading killer of African American women aged twenty-five to forty-four, accounting for roughly 11 per cent of all deaths in this demographic. That's why EJAF has invested heavily in projects around the United States that target African Americans as well as other communities that are still disproportionately impacted by AIDS.

Now, it's one thing to be in a major city with basic facilities. It's quite another to be sick and alone in the middle of nowhere. Frankly, I wonder if most Americans know how bad it is for some people in the rural South. Take Loretta. She was thirty-three years old and a single mother when she found out that she was HIV-positive. Her ex-husband had been incarcerated. She was already chronically depressed; with her HIV diagnosis, she was terrified of what would happen to her. Who would care for her three sons?

Loretta is like a lot of women in Southwest Louisiana. Young, African American, from a poor family. Many don't get the education they need, and many drop out of school, get married young, or have children while they're still teenagers. These women are at high risk for contracting HIV.

As recently as 2008, emergency rooms in Southwest Louisiana were clogging up with people admitted with late-stage AIDS. The scenes of emaciated people who had wasted away from the disease looked more like something you would expect to see in sub-Saharan Africa, not America. In an age when antiretrovirals are widely available in the richest country in the world, people were needlessly dying. They still are. It's no wonder that Loretta was paralysed with fear by her diagnosis.

In response to the crisis in Southwest Louisiana, Terry Estes, the executive director of the Southwest Louisiana AIDS Council (SLAC), and Dr Carlos Choucino, the medical director of the Comprehensive Care Clinic in Lake Charles, Louisiana, decided they needed to develop better ways to reach people living with HIV/AIDS. They learned from research that 'navigator' models, where people are guided to get access to comprehensive services, are very successful with AIDS patients. So, in 2008, SLAC and the Comprehensive Care Clinic partnered to identify patients throughout the region who needed access to care, especially in nearby rural areas.

Loretta was referred to SLAC and immediately connected with Angela Hursey, the organisation's health system navigator. Angela is an amazing woman, one of the many heroes doing battle on the front lines of the AIDS epidemic. She personally connects with every client who walks through the door, and she becomes a fierce advocate for his or her health and welfare. She believes in her clients, and in turn helps her clients to believe in themselves.

It's this sort of individual attention that makes all the difference. People living with AIDS often feel like statistics – and it's no wonder, because that is how they're treated most of the time. But at SLAC, Angela insists on treating her clients like human beings, with individual needs, concerns, challenges, and circumstances. This sounds simple and obvious, yet it's all too rare in health-care settings. I can relate to the need for individual attention and care, because that was what really helped me to get clean and to stay sober. Being treated with dignity, with compassion, like a real person with individual struggles, is what empowered me to turn my life around.

Whenever someone like Loretta walks into SLAC, Angela's first order of business is to get the person immediate access to care. She will literally take her clients to the hospital screening office so they can figure out what kind of financial assistance they might be able to get. She'll walk them to the lab to get tested. She'll go with them to their first doctor's appointment. She'll do whatever it takes to get them to take control of their health. If they stop going to their appointments or taking their medication, she'll pick them back up and walk them through the process all over again. After her clients are stable, she'll hand them over to a medical case manager to keep track of their progress.

I have to pause for a moment to point something out. EJAF is thrilled to have SLAC as our grantee. And we're grateful for the many other philanthropists who help fund their work. But SLAC and other groups like them would not be able to operate without the funding and assistance provided by the Ryan White CARE Act. I am deeply touched, and grateful, that Ryan's name is attached to this extraordinary work.

And it really is extraordinary, and very much needed, because it's still the case that in communities across America people with AIDS are sometimes treated like dirt. If they're gay, it can be even worse. They're so afraid of the judgement of their communities, even their families, that they won't get tested. Despite how far we've come, people in America today still experience the abuses that Ryan suffered. That's why some HIV-positive people travel hours from their homes to get help from SLAC. The organisation works hard to make clients whose families have ostracised them feel safe.

Thanks to SLAC and its dedicated caseworkers like Angela, Loretta started managing her disease. She went back to school to finish her GED. Today, she volunteers with SLAC, facilitating a women's support group. She even has her own office space, where she mentors other people who are struggling to come to terms with HIV/AIDS.

Loretta is doing what Ryan did. She is taking her experience, her story, and sharing it with others. She is using it to help them get through this incredibly difficult experience. She's a living reminder that we cannot simply treat the disease; we must treat the person.

When confronted with an enormous crisis like AIDS, it's easy to feel helpless. And in the face of huge numbers – millions of people infected, billions of dollars spent – it's easy to feel, as an individual, or even as an organisation, that we can't make a difference. But SLAC is an example of how a relatively small amount of money can go a really long way when compassion is at the centre of our efforts.

This is true for all marginalised populations, everywhere. Take the formerly incarcerated, for instance. They are among the most marginalised populations in the United States. And the formerly incarcerated who are HIV-positive are even further marginalised.

In New York, after an HIV-positive prisoner finishes his sentence, he's whisked away from an upstate detention facility and dropped off at the Port Authority bus station in Manhattan. He's usually given no more than $50, three days of medication, and a list of social service organisations that might be able to help.

Imagine: You are standing all alone by the bus or the subway. You haven't been outside the walls of prison, let alone in the middle of Midtown, in years. You have nowhere to go, maybe no one to call. And the clock has started ticking – you have seventy-two hours until your medication runs out.

For Carl, after twenty-four years in prison, that experience made him feel like he was Rip van Winkle, waking up to a whole new world. Everybody around him was talking into a mobile phone. He had used a token the last time he rode the subway; what on earth was a MetroCard?

The world had changed, and so had Carl. He was infected with HIV in prison, and he left with AIDS.

Carl was luckier than many; someone he 'ran with' picked him up from the Port Authority. They spent the next three days driving around to every single organisation on the list he was given when he was released from prison. At all of these places, places that were supposed to help him, he heard the same thing: 'Where's your Medicaid card?'

Carl had been released without any documentation of his HIV status, and since he didn't have Medicaid, there were few places he could go to be tested. He waited hours at a city agency to apply for public assistance in order to get the funds he needed to buy medication, but there was a forty-five-day waiting period to determine if he was eligible for benefits.

Carl's story is all too common. The United States imprisons a higher percentage of its population than any other nation in the world: more than 2.3 million people, or 1 in every 104 adults. Almost a quarter of the world's prisoners are in America. And as of December 2008, about 1.5 per cent of all prisoners in the nation were HIV-positive. When these HIV-positive prisoners re-enter society, very few are connected with services to give them stability and support while they figure out how to handle their health and their new lives.

That was the case for Carl. He was overwhelmed, exhausted, and almost totally defeated when he showed up late in the afternoon at Bailey House, a halfway house in East Harlem for people living with HIV/AIDS. By the time he walked through the front door, he was out of medication and he was a ball of anxiety. That's when Carl met Chris Olin, a caseworker for Project FIRST at Bailey House – another real-life hero. Chris is one of those exceptional people. You know, those people who just immediately put you at ease. Chris said to Carl, 'I've got this for you.'

It can be paralysing to be in the throes of your own crisis. I remember that feeling when I walked into rehab, like I had no control over anything that was happening to me, like I didn't know where to begin. When I was told not to worry, when I was told that people were going to help me, it was like an enormous weight lifted off my chest. Suddenly I had a chance to get better, because I wasn't alone any more.

I imagine that's how Carl felt when he met Chris. It was the first moment in a long time, maybe ever, that Carl had been treated with such dignity. That his anxiety, the trauma in his life, had been acknowledged. That somebody had his back and said, 'I'm with you.' That's when everything changed for Carl.

Project FIRST stands for Formerly Incarcerated

Rental Support and Training, and it's a programme run by Bailey House to support HIV-positive ex-offenders who are homeless or in danger of becoming homeless. It helps people like Carl with whatever they need to get back on their feet, to stay healthy, and to stay out of trouble. Within the first few weeks, Project FIRST connects their clients with a rental assistance programme run by the City of New York. Because of the flexible funding that EJAF and others provide, Bailey House is able to cover necessities such as security deposits and first month's rent, so that clients can get into safe housing immediately. After all, if you don't have anywhere to lay your head at night, how are you going to get the rest of your life together?

My foundation has been supporting this project at Bailey House since 2007, and we couldn't be happier with how far they've come. Since Project FIRST got off the ground in 2003, they have successfully placed more than two hundred people in permanent housing, and they have also connected them to the care they need to ensure their health and well-being. Many are still in the same apartments.

To me, Project FIRST is a tremendously efficient weapon against the AIDS crisis in New York City. We know that ex-offenders leave prison with dispro-portionately high rates of HIV. We know that they often don't have a way to get the medical care they need, let alone a place to live. We know that their lack of job opportunities makes it all the more likely that they could slip back into risky sex, drug abuse, and other behaviour that would put them in danger of spreading the disease or land them back in detention. Common sense says, let's address all of these problems quickly – let's not be afraid to help the very people who need the most help. Let's not let stigma get in the way.

One of the things I love most about Project FIRST is that the programme does more than fight AIDS; it helps people in the most basic ways. Caseworkers like Chris walk clients through the system and show them how to do everyday things such as open a bank account and figure out where they can go grocery shopping. They help clients get back into the community, find a doctor, take their medications regularly, get vocational training, and start taking care of themselves. For instance, Chris connected Carl with a clinic where he could go for medical tests, treatment, and medications, and Chris also got the necessary documentation of Carl's AIDS status and income level to qualify him for housing assistance.

People who go through Bailey House's programme have much better health outcomes. And they are far less likely to end up back in the penal system. Typically, more than 40 per cent of U.S. prisoners wind up returning to state prison within the first three years of being released. Fewer than 10 per cent of Bailey House beneficiaries are reincarcerated.

A few months after meeting Chris, Carl walked back into Bailey House looking like he had just come off a golf course. The angry, anxious, and desperate ex-offender was now a dapper, healthy, employed man, wearing Bermuda shorts and a polo shirt, supporting himself, managing his HIV, and in a relationship with a woman he met at Bailey House. Today, Carl is mentoring fellow ex-offenders and doing peer outreach to get others living with HIV into care. He also testifies in front of the New York State Parole Board about the value of programmes such as Bailey House's. It's no wonder that he's willing to do so much for the organisation. As Carl has said many times, 'Chris and Bailey House saved my life.'

The Elton John AIDS Foundation has funded hundreds of projects. Each one operates a bit differently. Each does different work for different populations. But every project we fund has one thing in common: it is committed to a compassionate response and to fighting the stigma that spreads HIV/AIDS. The organisations target their work to the most marginalised populations, those who most need the services but are least likely to get them. They advocate against policies that promote discrimination. They shine a light on the taboo subjects that nobody wants to talk about but that have everything to do with this horrible disease. Most of all they treat each person they see in a holistic way.

That term, 'holistic,' is thrown around a lot in medical circles. You hear doctors talking about caring for the whole patient, seeing to all of his or her medical needs at once. With HIV/AIDS, as with most diseases, it's more than just the way the body itself works. So many people with the virus are also poor and vulnerable. They often need shelter, food, mental health services, employment opportunities, and people to care for and support them. They need critical help at critical moments to ensure their disease doesn't come to define, or end, their lives.

It's crucial to treat every single person – regardless of background or circumstance or HIV status – as a whole person, as an individual with dreams to fulfil and goals to achieve. When we treat people as worthy of love, their worth is realised for all the world to see. Ultimately, this is the most powerful weapon we have against stigma, and indeed against AIDS.

Whether you are the richest man alive or you have absolutely nothing, you deserve to be treated with dignity and compassion. That is the insight that inspires the work of my foundation. And that, I have come to believe, is how we will end AIDS.

8

A Great Power

Every now and again, someone will ask if I get nervous on stage. Or they'll want to know about the most intimidating audience I've ever played to. At this point in my career, I've been lucky to perform at some of the world's most extraordinary venues, sometimes for audiences of half a million people. Every time I walk out on stage it's not nerves that I feel but the thrill of performing and the excitement of the crowd. I still love it after all these years. But there was one stage that made me nervous beyond belief. One audience that was more intimidating than any other. It wasn't a stadium concert with a sea of screaming fans. I can't ever recall being more nervous than on the day when I testified before the United States Senate.

It had been a decade since I created the foundation. As I said before, our intention was never to become one of the biggest AIDS organisations in the world – far from it. We were simply trying to help people in need. But, sadly, the need never ended; it grew steadily with each passing year. And so, in 2002, after ten years of doing this work, I had become – much to my surprise – a voice people listened to on the subject of fighting AIDS.

That's how I was summoned one day to Washington. I got word through EJAF that Senator Ted Kennedy intended to hold a hearing on the state of the AIDS epidemic and the international response to it, as part of his effort to increase funding for treatment programmes around the world. He planned to invite several witnesses to educate the Senate Health, Education, Labor, and Pensions Committee on the disease, and to make the case for a new appropriation of money. His office asked me to be one of them. I was deeply honoured by the invitation. And, from that moment on, I was extremely nervous as well.

I still remember our car driving up Pennsylvania Avenue toward Capitol Hill. I don't care how many times you see the U.S. Capitol Building; each and every time it is simply breath-taking. There's something about the way it was built, its very design, that exudes power and influence, and reminds you of the extraordinary history contained within.

Our car turned onto Constitution Avenue and headed up toward the Russell Senate Office Building. We got out and were greeted by a member of Ted Kennedy's staff – and a dozen reporters. We rushed quickly past them and into the grandeur of a Washington icon. The archways and columns. The marble statues. The awe-inspiring rotunda that echoed the noise of our shoes as we walked, adding a pointed sound of purpose to each step. We followed the staffer up one of two sweeping marble staircases. 'We're going to have breakfast and a small reception in the Caucus Room,' she told us. 'There are a lot of senators looking forward to meeting you.'

The Caucus Room, I was told, has an impressive history all its own. When the *Titanic* sank, this was where they held hearings to investigate what went wrong. It's where the Army–McCarthy hearings were held and where the Watergate hearings took place as well. And for reasons I swear I will never understand, it's where I was welcomed for a breakfast held in my honour. The room itself is something to behold. Pilasters from floor to ceiling in the classic Corinthian style. Imposing red curtains with gold fringe, draped across three massive windows. Century-old chandeliers and a ceiling with exceptional detail. It was enough to intimidate anyone, more than enough to intimidate me. And that was before I realised who was standing inside.

Senator Kennedy made a beeline toward me. We had never met before, but he shook my hand with both of his and embraced me as an old friend might. I've met a lot of famous people in my day, but shaking Ted Kennedy's hand was like touching history. He was a political icon from one of the most important families in America. The brother of President John F. Kennedy and of U.S. senator and attorney general Bobby Kennedy. A former presidential candidate himself and an extraordinary statesman. I wasn't sure what to say to such a man, but he instantly put me at ease.

The next thing I knew, I was shaking hands with Senator Orrin Hatch. Now, it's probably easy to imagine my not being a particularly big fan of Senator Hatch. He is an extremely conservative Republican from Utah, and we disagree on just about every issue I can imagine. But after Ryan's death, it was Senator Hatch who pushed for the Ryan White CARE Act. It was Senator Hatch who, with his friend Senator Kennedy, authored the bill. And it was the two of them together who ensured that the bill made it through Congress with bipartisan support. And so, in truth, as I stood there shaking Senator Hatch's hand, with Senator Kennedy just behind me, I was surrounded by AIDS heroes, by people who had used the power of their station to save millions of lives.

I met several other senators and members of Congress

before sitting down for breakfast, and I saw a few familiar faces, too. The International AIDS Trust was hosting the breakfast, and Sandy Thurman, my friend and its president, was there to greet me. Sandy is a legend in the AIDS advocacy community, and because she was based in Atlanta, I knew her well. In 1997, she had been named the director of the Office of National AIDS Policy at the White House by President Bill Clinton, a fitting choice for that critical job. She, too, would be testifying.

Deborah Dortzbach, the international director of the HIV/AIDS programmes for World Relief, was there as well. Our organisation had worked quite closely with hers. And there were others, also testifying, whom I knew by reputation but hadn't had a chance to meet until then. Dr Peter Mugyenyi, one of the world's most respected AIDS specialists, had come all the way from Kampala, Uganda, where he founded and directed a clinical research centre. Also present was a relentless advocate for women's health during the AIDS crisis, Dr Allan Rosenfield, the legendary dean of the Mailman School of Public Health at Columbia University.

These were, without question, some of the most respected leaders in the fight against AIDS. And there I was, a bit dumbfounded to be among them.

The outpouring of support I felt that day was

remarkable. It contrasted starkly with the early days of the disease, when fear and stigma kept AIDS deep in the shadows of American life. Here we were, many years later, in one of the most powerful places on earth, talking about what we could do to fight the disease together. I was very moved.

After breakfast, I was escorted by Ted Kennedy back to his office, where we were joined by Senator Hatch, Senator Patrick Leahy, Senator Bill Frist, and Senator Hillary Clinton for a candid conversation about how much money it would take to truly combat AIDS globally and what strategies we could employ to get it done. The perspectives in the room were amazing. These were not only U.S. senators; they were also leading experts in the fight against AIDS. In 1981, Bill Frist was a third-year surgical resident in Boston when reports of the disease started surfacing. To that point, doctors had considered blood to be mostly sterile; suddenly they knew it could be deadly. Frist had to radically alter his surgical procedures. Double gloves during surgery and eye protection. In the very early days, before there was treatment of any kind, Frist wouldn't make his assistants scrub in to work on an AIDS patient if they were afraid to; that's how little was known about the HIV virus then, how much fear persisted even in the medical community.[1]

Then there was Senator Clinton, who had travelled the globe as First Lady during the height of the AIDS crisis. She knew well that, by 2002, the AIDS epidemic abroad was very different from the one unfolding at home. She knew the stakes, because she had seen the effects herself. I was struck by how incredibly well educated all of the senators were on the crisis. Each and every one of them really knew what he or she was talking about. I was humbled by their respect for me and my work, their recognition that I wasn't just a rock star with a hobby. They were interested in my perspective, and I was honoured to share it with this group of distinguished leaders.

I had, by that point, got control of my nerves. The warmth I was shown certainly helped. And a good thing, too, because moments later, a staffer knocked on the door. 'Senator,' he said to Kennedy, 'it's time.'

The hearing room was smaller, but no less grand, than the Caucus Room. And it was absolutely packed with people. By then, I had broken off from the senators and was ushered down the aisle to a table up front, where those of us testifying would sit. As soon as I sat down in front of my name placard, I was surrounded by photo-journalists. How surreal that moment was. I'm no stranger to cameras, but there was something about the context that made it all feel very different. I was about to perform, but the stakes were higher than they'd ever been.

Above the flashing cameras I saw the senators enter the chamber and begin filling in the dais. 'The hearing will come to order,' said Ted Kennedy, who chaired the committee. The room fell quiet. 'We welcome our guests this morning, who bring to this issue the challenges that we are facing in international AIDS, a wealth of experience and an extraordinary sense of compassion, and a series of recommendations about how we as a country can be even more effective in giving this the kind of world priority that it deserves.'

Senator Kennedy then recognised his colleagues, who one by one gave their opening statements, each more poignant than the last. When they were finished, we were told that we had just about an hour for our testimony and that there would be questions from the senators after our statements. Sandy gave her statement first. It was beautiful, profoundly important, and extremely compelling.

Then it was my turn.

I thanked Senator Kennedy and the others for this honour – for asking my opinion, especially as a British man. And then I began to read from remarks I had prepared.

'I've worn many hats in my career, but the hat of

policy maker is not one of them,' I said. 'I will not take up your time to tell you facts and numbers you already know. Instead, I will tell you how I feel.'

I told them that it had been twelve years since we had lost Ryan White, how devastating it had been, but how extraordinary Congress's reaction to Ryan's death had been as well. 'The month Ryan died,' I said, 'this committee passed the Ryan White CARE Act that dramatically increased funding for care and treatment of people with AIDS. Mr Chairman, the rest of the world looks at this legislation as a sign of what America can do for its people. We are here today to explore what America can do for the world.'

I then tried to give them a sense of what my foundation had been able to accomplish internationally, the kind of projects we were funding, the kind of difference, in small ways, we were making. I told them about an AIDS hospice in Soweto, South Africa, that we'd established. 'Among people with AIDS, the greatest fear is not the fear of dying,' I told them, 'but the fear of dying alone. At our hospice, no one dies alone.

'But, Mr Chairman, our hospice in South Africa has eight beds, and the nation has more than four million people infected with HIV. We are doing everything we can with what we have, and we have comforted many people and saved many lives. But we have not done nearly enough. The people on the front lines fighting this disease need reinforcements, and they need them now.'

I called on Congress to increase funding for education and prevention, for voluntary testing and counselling, for care for those who were dying of AIDS, and for orphans.

'If the world is going to make a significant, decisive intervention to change the course of this pandemic, it's going to have to start here. And it might as well start now,' I said. 'When Ryan White was asked by a reporter if he had a message for medical researchers working on AIDS, he said, "Hurry up." We all need to hurry up. Every day we delay, we lose more lives, and we lose a little more of our humanity.'

The point I wanted to drive home was not only the urgency. It was the possibility. There really was something the United States could be doing, something profound. That is, if it chose to. This wasn't a case of wanting to solve an unsolvable problem. Millions of lives were on the line, and millions could be saved by the U.S. government.

'It's true that one nation cannot defeat AIDS in two hundred nations,' I admitted. 'But two hundred nations cannot defeat AIDS without the help of one. This one. If the U.S. does little, other nations will see in that an excuse to do little. If the United States does a lot, other nations will do a lot, because they will see in your resolve a new hope of victory. When the United States fights, it wins.'

With that, and a few more thank-yous, I concluded my remarks. I took a deep breath, inhaled the scene around me, and hoped that, just maybe, something I had said would make a difference, if only a small one.

When the hearing was over, Senator Kennedy invited us back to his office for a private gathering. The walls were lined with pictures of his famous brothers. It was a reminder that history is made by the people who stand up to make it. We walked outside on his balcony overlooking the Capitol and took it all in. I thought about what had happened that day, but more than that, I thought about what might happen tomorrow. I thought about the future, the next battle lines to be drawn in the fight against AIDS.

Senator Chris Dodd and a few others who had testified stood out there with us, and Senator Dodd thanked us for our commitment to ridding the world of the disease. During my testimony I had said that, while I wasn't a student of American government, it was my understanding that there were two sides of Pennsylvania Avenue, and only one end – Congress – was in charge of the money. That it was up to them to take up the fight.

Senator Dodd had responded from the dais in jest, 'Tell that to the other end.' He meant that I should press my case with President George W. Bush at the White House, of course.

But as it turned out, I wouldn't need to do any such thing. Just nine months later, everything changed when, on 28 January 2003, President Bush gave his second State of the Union address.

I had never been a fan of the second President Bush. I found his worldview to be totally warped. I thought the values he claimed to uphold didn't match his policies. I thought his rhetoric against gay marriage, against civil unions, really against any expansion of gay rights at all, was deeply harmful and homophobic. Needless to say, I was not looking forward to watching the speech.

But I planned to watch it anyway. I'd lived part-time in the United States for many years at that point, and it felt to me, even though I was a British citizen, that I had an obligation to hear what the president had to say, even if I expected to disagree. And, in fact, I disagreed with almost all of it. This was the speech, you may recall, where Bush made his case for going to war in Iraq. It was the speech where he claimed that there was a grave threat of weapons of mass destruction from Saddam Hussein, and that in the name of the 'war on terror' we had to act swiftly.

Still, I remember that speech not because of what was said about Iraq or terrorism or abortion or taxes. I remember it for what President Bush said about AIDS:

Today, on the continent of Africa, nearly 30 million people have the AIDS virus, including 3 million children under the age of 15. There are whole countries in Africa where more than one-third of the adult population carries the infection. More than 4 million require immediate drug treatment. Yet across that continent, only 50,000 AIDS victims – only 50,000 – are receiving the medicine they need.

I couldn't believe what I was hearing. The president of the United States, standing in front of a joint session of Congress, was calling attention to the crisis we had spent more than a decade fighting. I knew the statistics he cited. I'd cited them myself hundreds of times.

'AIDS can be prevented,' he implored. 'Antiretroviral drugs can extend life for many years. And the cost of those drugs has dropped from $12,000 a year to under $300 a year, which places a tremendous possibility within our grasp.'

At that point, as if I were watching a football game, my heart was racing. 'Ladies and gentlemen,' Bush continued, 'seldom has history offered a greater opportunity to do so much for so many. We have confronted, and will continue to confront, HIV/AIDS in our own country. And to meet a severe and urgent crisis abroad, tonight I propose the Emergency Plan for AIDS Relief, a work of mercy beyond all current international efforts to help the people of Africa.'

Then, he told us the numbers. I can't overstate what a big moment this was:

> This comprehensive plan will prevent 7 million new AIDS infections, treat at least 2 million people with life-extending drugs, and provide humane care for millions of people suffering from AIDS and for children orphaned by AIDS. I ask the Congress to commit $15 billion over the next five years, including nearly $10 billion in new money, to turn the tide against AIDS in the most afflicted nations of Africa and the Caribbean.

This was the moment when funding the global fight against AIDS became a question of 'billions' instead of 'millions.' It's hard to put into perspective just how huge it was. But this should give you an idea: Just four years earlier, we had considered it a tremendous victory – we actually celebrated – when President Clinton had convinced Congress to increase global AIDS spending from $125 million to $225 million. This was more than sixty times that amount.

Indeed, President Bush's global AIDS initiative, which became known as the President's Emergency Plan for AIDS Relief, or PEPFAR, was the largest commitment by any nation to combat a global disease in history. The $15 billion was to be spent in just a five-year period, from 2003 to 2008. And when it was renewed in 2008, that number more than tripled to $48 billion, an extraordinary sum.

Congress responded to the president's request. Many of the same senators I had met with and testified before were instrumental in passing PEPFAR. The results, thanks to their efforts and President Bush's commitment, have been breath-taking: According to the U.S. State Department, which administers PEPFAR, the United States has given almost 4 million men, women, and children around the world access to antiretroviral treatment. It supported HIV testing and counselling for nearly 10 million pregnant women in 2011 alone. And because PEPFAR got antiretrovirals into the hands of more than 660,000 HIV-positive pregnant women, America was able to ensure that some 200,000 infants were born *without* the disease. Thirteen million people received care and support through PEPFAR in 2011, and 40 million received testing or counselling. President

Bush's decision to take aggressive action has, without question, saved *millions* of lives.

PEPFAR also meant that EJAF-UK and other non-profit organisations could look at dramatically expanding their work in Africa. Because the drugs and much of the infrastructure was to be paid for under PEPFAR, EJAF could find smart ways of scaling up programmes for women and children infected with HIV from the hundreds to now the hundreds of thousands. I have met dozens of these beneficiaries: pregnant women whose babies will live their lives HIV-free.

Of course, PEPFAR's creation and implementation was not without controversy. PEPFAR explicitly excluded certain populations, including sex workers, which is both intolerable and illogical. As I've written here many times, you cannot win a war if you refuse to fight it on certain battlefields. There was also controversy around the requirement by PEPFAR that significant funds be spent on abstinence-only educational programmes, which are a complete waste of money, since they've been proven to be marginally effective at best. It would be far better to spend those resources on treatment and also on prevention programmes that actually work. But, taken on the whole, the impact of PEPFAR is truly staggering. It was, and today continues to be, the single greatest assault on HIV/AIDS since the disease emerged.

There were lessons to be learned in watching liberal Democrats and conservative Republicans come together to make PEPFAR a reality. The first, and one of the most important, is that you cannot assume the worst in people. Instead, it may be possible, more times than you'd think, to work with someone on a shared goal. To find common ground. To achieve great things through unlikely partnerships.

It was easy for me to despise President Bush from afar, to assume, wrongly, that he would never be an ally in any fight I was involved in. The truth, it turned out, was quite different. I learned this during the creation of PEPFAR in 2003, and again in 2004, when I finally had the opportunity to meet him.

I was very surprised and flattered to be selected to receive the prestigious Kennedy Center Honors, which are given to only a few entertainers each year in recognition of their cultural contributions to American life. It is a big deal – I knew that much. But to be quite honest, at the time, David and I were torn about whether I should accept the honour. The award itself is presented by the sitting president of the United States, and I was no great fan of George W. Bush, apart from his position on AIDS. More than that, I was morally opposed to many of his policies, and I took personal offence at many of his pronouncements. Ultimately, however, David and I came to realise that the Kennedy Center Honors were bestowed not by a president but by a nation, and my love and respect for America were much more important than any political statement I could make by refusing to accept an award from George W. Bush.

David and I flew to Washington, and the first order of business was a formal dinner at the U.S. State Department, during which each Kennedy Center honoree is presented with a medallion. After a few kind words, Colin Powell, the secretary of state, hung the medallion around my neck. When I got back to my seat, David and I chuckled to ourselves, because as it turns out the medallion itself is several metal bars attached to a big, rainbow-coloured ribbon that looks identical to the gay-pride flag. And I was very proud to wear it, of course.

The next day, we went to the White House for the formal citation reading ceremony. As we walked up those grand steps, it wasn't excitement we felt but apprehension. We were entering the lion's den, we thought. David and I had no idea how we would be treated or what the experience would be like for a same-sex couple visiting a Republican White House that seemed openly hostile to gays. But we were immediately put at ease by an Air Force pilot who was assigned to be our White House escort. You've never seen a more handsome man in your life, especially in that uniform! And what's more, I instantly knew he was gay. These were the days when you weren't supposed to 'ask,' and they weren't supposed to 'tell.' But, of course, I couldn't help myself. 'You're gay, aren't you?' I said. He smiled and nodded. To this day, our Air Force escort is a great friend of ours.

The award presentation was in one of the beautifully ornate receiving rooms at the White House. President Bush read citations for each honoree. When it came to my turn, the president began to list some of my hit songs over the years, including 'Crocodile Rock,' 'Daniel,' and – in one of the president's legendary verbal miscues – 'Bernie and the Jets.' Just then, First Lady Laura Bush interrupted the president and yelled out, 'It's "*Bennie* and the Jets"!'

The president and everyone in the audience had quite a laugh. That is, except Dick Cheney. When President Bush finished reading my citation and the audience applauded, David and I were stunned to see the vice president sitting there with his arms folded and a scowl on his face. It may have been that he still had raw feelings about my quote to a British publication a few weeks prior, that 'Bush and this administration are the worst thing that has ever happened to America.' I suppose I can't blame him for being unhappy with me about that!

That evening, there was a wonderful gala concert at the Kennedy Center Opera House – a very moving event during which my friends Billy Joel and Kid Rock serenaded me with my own songs. David and I sat in a special box with my fellow awardees: Warren Beatty, Ossie Davis and Ruby Dee, Joan Sutherland, and John Williams. At intermission, our group filed into the hospitality area behind the box. Our seats were next to the president's, and little did I realise that our boxes shared this hospitality room in common. Suddenly I was standing next to a bunch you wouldn't think of as my usual concert-goers: Donald Rumsfeld, Dick Cheney, Condoleezza Rice, Colin Powell, and, yes, President Bush.

It was a surprising moment indeed, but the real surprise would come when the president and I had a chance to speak. I remember having the greatest conversation with him. He was warm, charming, and very complimentary, not only about my music but also about the work of my foundation. He knew all about what we were doing, and he was endlessly knowledgeable about HIV/AIDS as well.

President Bush and I discussed the epidemic for quite

a while, and he asked if there was anything he could do to help EJAF. I thanked him for his offer, but I said that his commitment to PEPFAR had already done a world of good, and I commended him for all he was doing to fight AIDS abroad. At that point, I felt compelled to ask if there was anything I could do to help him. 'Yeah,' he said, with a look of dead seriousness on his face. 'Tell the French they need to give more money.'

You see, at that point, France had not yet made a significant commitment to fighting the global AIDS epidemic, and President Bush was truly angry about it. The French government has since spearheaded the creation of a wonderful multi-government programme called UNITAID, which funds the purchase of HIV/ AIDS medication and other global health needs for poor countries through a small tax on the purchase of airline tickets. But back in 2004, President Bush was lobbying for them to do more. This wasn't a political issue to him, or some side project. He genuinely cared about people around the world who were dying of AIDS.

I'll never forget our meeting that night. President Bush and I haven't seen each other or talked since, and like many people, I deeply regretted much of what he did in office, especially the wars he waged in Iraq and

Afghanistan. But my encounter with George W. Bush reminded me not to rush to judgement about people, especially when it comes to fighting AIDS. More than anything, we need allies in this fight, not enemies.

That was one important lesson learned from the implementation of PEPFAR. The other was one I grew to understand, not just from watching PEPFAR's creation but from my own experience testifying before Congress, and from years of EJAF's work around the world: there is no institution on earth, not one, that is as capable of making sweeping changes as government.

Governments have the power to entirely remake the societies they govern. They have the power to battle, to wage war, not just on other nations but on poverty, on injustice, on epidemics. They have the resources and influence to change the future, and the choice of whether or not to do so. And with a disease such as AIDS in particular, they have a unique ability to fund treatment and care, education and prevention. They can ensure that all their citizens have access to life-saving medicine. Governments are, without question, the single biggest factor in determining whether AIDS will be a death sentence for their people, or whether their HIV-positive citizens will survive.

Governments of the world are more than just resources for funding. They also have an unmatched ability, without spending a penny, to fight the terrible torment of stigma. Government, after all, has the ultimate megaphone. All it takes is a president or a prime minister to say, 'It doesn't matter who you are or where you come from, you deserve the dignity of having your life valued as much as the rest of us.' All it takes is for lawmakers to speak up for their marginalised constituents. All it takes is leaders to proclaim they will not let a disease ravage people living in their communities. In an age of ubiquitous communications, these statements alone can have a tremendous impact.

This is a sunny analysis of the power of government, but there is also a darker reality at work, and one I must acknowledge. Government has extraordinary power for good, but it can also be the world's greatest impediment to change. Governments can decide to make homosexuality illegal, to force people to stay, by law, in the closet. Governments can decide that needle exchange, however effective it may be, is just too loathsome a concept, that if the disease must spread through and kill drug users, then so be it. Governments can choose to act, and they can also choose not to. More often than not, the latter is the case.

In some ways, this is what foundations like mine have the hardest time overcoming. There are places around the world where we want to help, where we have the resources to help, but the obstacles of government are far too great. Too often, we aren't able to reach the people who most need our assistance. How can you get the treatment you need when coming out into the open can lead to criminal punishment? The answer, all over the world, is that you can't.

That is why perhaps the biggest stumbling block we face in our effort to eradicate AIDS is the prevalence of governmental backwardness.

Look at India, for example, the world's second-most populous country. Homosexuality was made illegal there by British colonial law in 1861. It was decriminalised, finally, in a 2009 ruling by the New Delhi high court, a ruling that is currently being appealed to India's Supreme Court. In the meantime, other courts have chosen to ignore the ruling. Men are still going to jail for having sex with other men.

This is both horrifically bigoted and hugely problematic from an institutional perspective. Gay men with HIV/AIDS in India must fear for their liberty when they seek treatment; a lot of them, as a result, choose not to get help. And so the disease spreads. The damage of homophobic laws is only compounded when political leaders choose to use their bully pulpit to spew hatred. This we saw in India in 2011, when the nation's health minister told an HIV/AIDS conference that he believed sex between men was 'unnatural.' 'Unfortunately,' he told the audience, 'there is this disease in the world and in this country where men are having sex with other men, which is completely unnatural and shouldn't happen, but it does.'[2]

This was an unspeakably inappropriate comment to make to any audience, by any person, but when you consider that this man was a national health minister, and the audience he was speaking to was a group of people trying to combat HIV in his country, it becomes all the more outrageous. There are 2.5 million people infected with HIV in India, and their government has said essentially, 'We don't care about *any* of you because *some* of you are gay.'

The irony is that as the health minister continued to speak, he illuminated one of the central points I've been making, one that people like him are largely responsible for causing. 'In our country,' he said, 'the numbers of men having sex with men are substantial, but it is very difficult to find them.' Difficult, of course, because homosexuality in India is still, for all intents and purposes, illegal.

We will never eradicate this disease when governments use their power so destructively, when they codify stigma and then spread it. Nor will we eradicate AIDS until governments understand the fundamental truth about the populations they govern: there is no 'other.' They might like to think about the groups they marginalize – drug users, gay men, people of colour, the poor – as somehow living segregated lives. But communities don't work like that. We all interact with one another, even when we don't know it. We do business with each other. We live next to one another. Oh, and by the way, yes, we have sex with each other. And so the idea that we can ignore marginalised populations – that we can let them retreat into the shadows to die and that doing so, morality aside, won't have any impact on the rest of the community – is as shamefully stupid as it is tragic.

When AIDS is ravaging drug users, it matters for those who don't use drugs. When AIDS is racing through the gay community, it matters for those who aren't gay. There is no 'other,' and if governments keep treating the disease as an 'other' problem, we will fail to end this epidemic.

One of the most heart-breaking examples of government stupidity is unfolding right now in Ukraine. As I mentioned, Ukraine is a nation where the disease is moving at a terrifying pace through the population. It is also a place where, recently, the government made a terrible choice, one that very well might result in the deaths of many Ukrainians.

Earlier, I told the story of the Lavra Clinic in Kiev, a wonderful institution that is one of the few lifelines for people living with HIV/AIDS in Ukraine. This extraordinary clinic is regarded by gay men in that country as the only safe place they can go to get treatment. And now, as I write this, it has been ordered to close by Ukraine's government.

You see, the clinic is adjacent to the historic Kiev-Pechersk Lavra monastery. The land the clinic sits on is owned by the monastery, and the monks there have apparently decided they no longer want the clinic next door. In June 2011, Ukraine's prime minister approved an order to close the clinic. Of all the land in Ukraine, they chose the location of the Lavra Clinic to make way for a luxury hotel.

The government claims that they will just relocate the facility, but no one at the clinic – not the doctors nor the patients – has been told where it will be moved. And at the time of the government's order to shutter the facility, the clinic hadn't been relocated at all. Keep in mind that even a modest delay in treatment could spell death for patients who depend on the Lavra Clinic's support. It's unclear at this point if the government has any intention of opening the clinic elsewhere. What is clear is the following: since Lavra is the most important HIV treatment centre in Ukraine, if its services are suspended or closed, people are going to get sick and die.

I've been to Ukraine many times, because EJAF funds a number of programmes there. I've seen firsthand the extraordinary life-saving services that clinics in Ukraine provide. And so, in November 2011, I returned to Kiev as part of a desperate campaign to turn things around. At a press conference, I'd had it. 'For fuck's sake, Ukraine!' I yelled for all who could hear it. 'You live in the twenty-first century, not the nineteenth century! This is a disgrace! It's a disgrace how some human beings are treated in this country!'

In the months since the order to close the clinic was handed down, EJAF has done everything it can to help raise awareness. Thanks to the protests of AUKN, Lavra's clients and supporters, EJAF, and many others, the debate is ongoing as to the ultimate fate of the Lavra Clinic. We're heartened that it seems we've been able to delay to this point the eviction of Lavra's patients.

But when it comes to the larger fight against AIDS in Ukraine, we are not naive. We are fighting a losing battle there, not because the disease is too strong but because it has the government as its accomplice.

Ukraine is one of the few countries in the region to acknowledge its AIDS crisis. Backsliding now, sending a message that people who are at risk of contracting

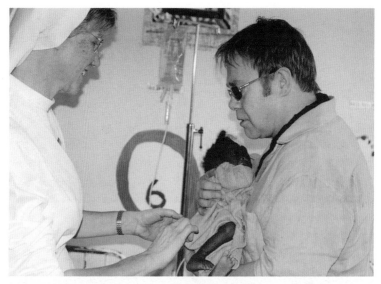

Discussing the prognosis for a baby with AIDS in rural South Africa. *(Sydney Duval)*

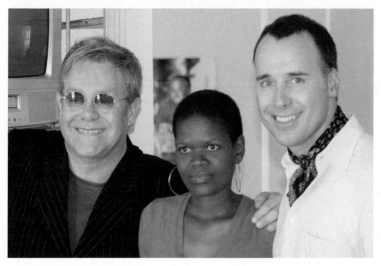

With Fumana and David in 2008 at the Simelela Rape Crisis Centre in Khayelit-sha, South Africa. Simelela is a twenty-four-hour, seven-day-a-week acute care centre that provides services to survivors of rape, the first of its kind in South Africa. Since being treated at the Simelela center, Fumana has devoted herself to rape survivor advocacy. *(Polly Steele)*

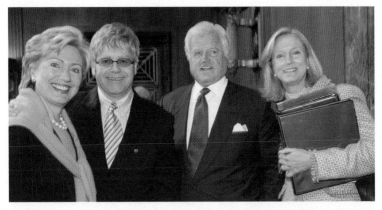

Senator Hillary Clinton, Senator Ted Kennedy, Director of the Office of National AIDS Policy Sandy Thurman, and I meet before testifying at a Senate hearing on the state of the AIDS epidemic on April 11, 2002. *(Vivian Ronay / Retna Ltd. / Corbis)*

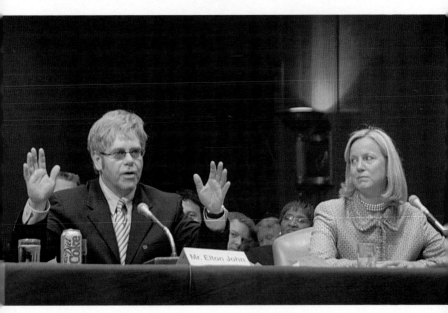

At the Senate hearing on April 11, 2002, with Sandy Thurman. In my testimonial, I said, "When Ryan White was asked by a reporter if he had a message for medical researchers working on AIDS, he said, 'Hurry up.' We all need to hurry up. Every day we delay, we lose more lives, and we lose a little more of our humanity." *(Vivian Ronay / Retna Ltd. / Corbis)*

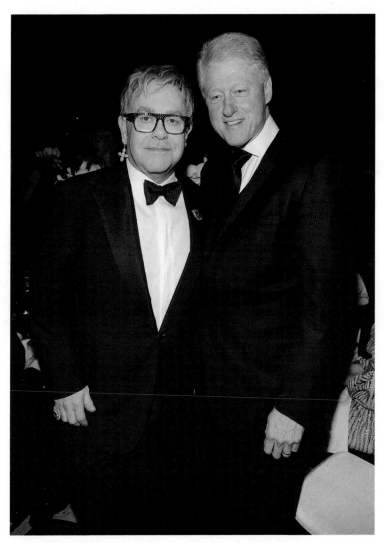

With former president Bill Clinton at EJAF's eighth annual benefit held on November 16, 2009, in New York City. EJAF honoured President Clinton that night with an Enduring Vision Award. The William J. Clinton Foundation has fought for the rights of those living with HIV/AIDS worldwide since 2002. *(Larry Busacca / WireImage / Getty Images)*

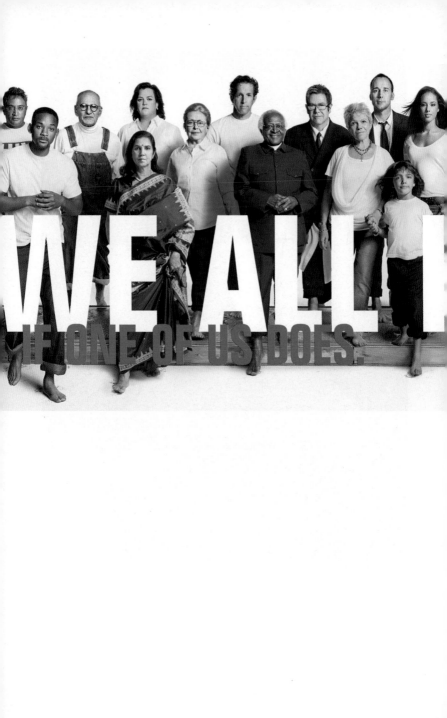

WE ALL

IF ONE OF US DOES.

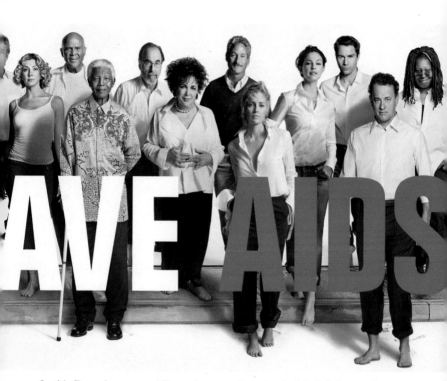

In this December 2005 public service campaign, shot by Mark Seliger and spearheaded by Kenneth Cole and KNOW HIV/AIDS, David and I joined other participants in demonstrating our commitment to the global fight against HIV/AIDS. *(Photograph by Mark Seliger)*

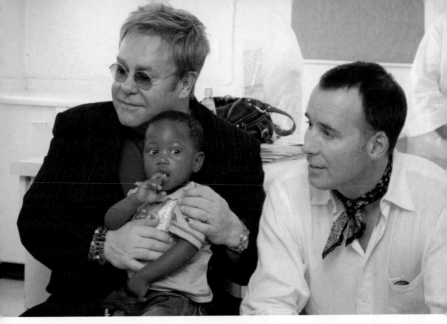

Holding a child at a mother-baby clinic in Cape Town, South Africa. EJAF-UK has helped more than 200,000 HIV-positive pregnant women in Africa to access medicine that protects their babies from acquiring HIV. *(Polly Steele)*

Holding baby Lev during a news conference at the state orphanage for children with HIV/AIDS in Makeyevka, Ukraine, on September 12, 2009. David and I were legally unable to adopt Lev from Ukraine, but the experience changed our lives by inspiring us to have a child. *(Handout / Reuters)*

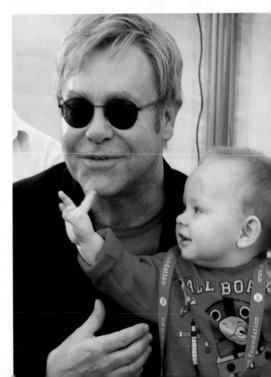

Visiting a state orphanage for children with HIV/AIDS in the town of Makeyevka, Ukraine, on September 12, 2009. EJAF first started working in Ukraine in 2002, funding an organisation that now supports more than 57,000 Ukrainians living with HIV/AIDS.
(© Gleb Garanich / Reuters)

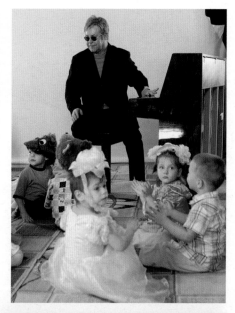

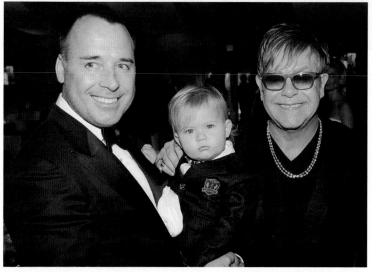

At EJAF's twentieth annual Academy Awards Viewing Party in West Hollywood on February 26, 2012. David and I have been together since 1993, and we are partners in everything, including the work of EJAF. Our beautiful son, Zachary, was born on Christmas Day, 2010. *(Larry Busacca / Getty Images)*

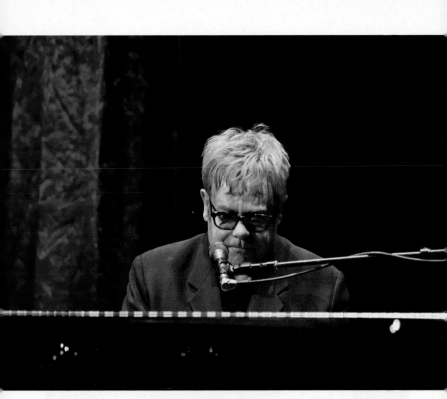

Performing at an event to celebrate the life and legacy of Ryan White in Indianapolis on April 28, 2010, marking twenty years since Ryan's death. He continues to inspire me each and every day. *(Nathaniel Edmunds Photography)*

HIV don't matter, will disastrously inflate the epidemic. The whole country will feel the effects of that. We know this because, tragically, it has happened in every other region where there is an HIV epidemic.

Government inaction will make Ukraine's already surging AIDS crisis even worse, full stop. And that will make the problem worse for *all* Ukrainians. Already the disease is spreading, out of the shadows, out of the drug dens. Further government inaction, obstruction, and delay are intolerable.

The point here is not just to condemn the Ukrainian government, though they certainly deserve it. The point is that unless governments treat all their citizens equally, we'll never end AIDS. That's the plain truth, no matter the continent or the context. It is as true in the West as it is in the developing world. It is true in poor countries and rich countries, in North America and North Africa. And so governments must make a choice. They can choose to spread stigma or they can choose to quash it. They can choose to spread treatment or instead spread bigotry and death. They can embrace the truth of this disease or they can continue to believe the lies they are telling themselves about HIV/AIDS and the people it affects.

Unfortunately, governments have a habit of lying not only to themselves but also to their people. I have been shocked at the misinformation that governments have spread, senselessly, at the direct cost of human life. But nothing I've seen in all my years of doing this work has shocked me more than the misinformation propagated by the government of South Africa.

It was in South Africa, several years ago, that President Thabo Mbeki became a leading voice among those known as AIDS denialists. In 2000, he spoke at the XIII International AIDS Conference in Durban and rejected all of the science we had learned about the disease to that point. He said that AIDS was caused by poverty, poor nourishment, poor health. He said it was the result of a failing immune system. And he said, emphatically, that it was not caused by a virus. As such, he concluded, it could not be treated with medicine. So he rejected free medicine for his people. He rejected grants for treatment and prevention programmes. He used the power he had been granted to stand between his citizens and efforts to save their lives.[3]

These were not abstract pronouncements by a fringe member of a government. These were the policies of a president – the leader of the nation. And the result, according to a Harvard paper published in 2008, was that 330,000 people died unnecessarily from the disease, and another 35,000 babies were born with it.[4] A quiet holocaust.

Mbeki was eventually ousted. Without him, South Africa has reversed itself, aiming to get treatment into the country as swiftly as possible. But the misinformation still lives on, not just in the minds of those who trusted the words of President Mbeki but also in the words of the new president, Jacob Zuma. When he was still the country's vice president, Zuma told South Africa that he'd had sex with an HIV-positive woman, but not to worry, he had taken a shower afterward to reduce his chance of contracting the illness.[5]

How many people, I wonder, have contracted the disease because they took Zuma's inexcusable advice to shower after unprotected sex?

I'm pleased to report that, as president, Zuma has mobilised more government support for the fight against AIDS in South Africa than any of his predecessors. But therein lies the great contradiction of government, and I'm not the first to point it out. The power to heal. The power to harm. Extraordinary power, and too often it is concentrated in the hands of those who don't understand the consequences of their deeds and words. And sometimes, the power is in the hands of truly evil people who just don't give a damn about human life.

This contradiction plays out not only in the developing world, not only in Eastern Europe and sub-

Saharan Africa, but also in the West. And, yes, even in the United States. *Especially* in the United States.

It might shock you to learn that in America today, thousands of low-income people are on government waiting lists to receive lifesaving HIV/AIDS medication that they cannot afford. These people are not necessarily poor. They are often either unemployed or work in jobs without health insurance and simply don't make enough to pay for their AIDS medication.

Consider the case of Steven Dimmick, a thirty-one-year-old man from Jacksonville, Florida. As the *Chicago Tribune* reported, he was forced to sell his car and his home, and he filed for bankruptcy protection in order to raise the cash for his HIV/AIDS treatment.[6] A federal effort called the AIDS Drug Assistance Program (ADAP) was designed to prevent people like Steven from falling through the cracks. But now waiting lists are swallowing them up. And make no mistake: the people on these lists will eventually die without treatment. Tragically, some have.

In 2011, more than 12,000 low-income, uninsured HIV-positive Floridians relied on ADAP to receive their medication. But many more needed help. Because Florida's ADAP program has been so severely underfunded, another 4,000 people sat on a waiting list for the treatment they needed to survive. Steven was one of these people. ADAP is a nationwide program, and at the time Florida had the largest waiting list of any state.

In 2011, Florida's governor, Rick Scott, sought deep budget cuts, and his administration proposed cost-saving changes to the state's ADAP program. The changes would have meant some 1,600 people who were receiving ADAP assistance would lose it. In June 2011, David and I wrote a letter to Governor Scott urging him to reconsider his administration's proposed changes to ADAP. We tried to explain to him what a lack of treatment would mean, not just for those living with the disease like Steven but for Florida and for the nation at large. We pleaded with him that 'denying HIV treatment to low-income people not only harms their health and increases the incidence of drug-resistant HIV, it also makes it more likely that these people can and will spread the disease to others.' David spoke to the Florida press. We wrote op-eds. We started an online petition and sent more than 4,000 signatures to Governor Scott.

The response we received was shocking. It was a letter from the Florida surgeon general, Dr Frank Farmer, written on the governor's stationery. It said, strangely, that because the waiting list for ADAP was so high, the Department of Health was considering new eligibility standards 'in an effort to ensure that Florida is allocating the dollars appropriated for AIDS drugs to those who are most vulnerable.' The implication, I suppose, being that there were people getting ADAP support who could afford to pay their own way. It was utter nonsense.

Dr Farmer defended the actions of Governor Scott's administration by suggesting that other states had taken similar cost-cutting steps. And then he had the audacity to close with the following: 'We cordially invite you to consider an ADAP fund-raising concert series in Florida. We would love to welcome you to the Sunshine State and I am confident your concerts will be a huge hit!'

A fucking benefit concert. As if that could raise anywhere *close* to the money needed to plug the gap. It was as condescending as it was completely idiotic. The American state of Florida, with its $69.1 *billion* annual budget, was proposing to outsource its AIDS efforts to a British musician. What a ludicrous idea, that a celebrity could be a substitute for a government. That really says it all, I think.

In the end, when the U.S. federal budget for 2011–2012 was passed, it included a $48 million increase for ADAP funds. It was enough to prevent Florida from making additional cuts. But it wasn't enough to cover thousands of people around the nation who, as I write this, continue to sit in desperation on waiting lists.

It is all too easy for political leaders to think about AIDS only in the abstract. It is all too easy for them to forget that there are real people counting on them for help, people who deserve the same chance to live a long life as anyone else.

In the end, the only way we will end AIDS is with a commitment to do so not just from *one* government but from *all* governments. A commitment from governors and presidents. From premiers and prime ministers. From Asia to Africa to Europe.

Governments can be the greatest force in the fight to rid the world of AIDS. But only if they so choose.

9

A Great Responsibility

About four months after President Bush announced PEPFAR in his State of the Union address, we were all feeling incredibly optimistic. Ten years into the foundation's creation, it really seemed as if, for the first time, we were on the verge of a breakthrough. The American government had made a historic commitment to ending AIDS. There was so much hope, so much adrenaline. It made me think of Ryan a lot. I guess many things do, but during those days, when it seemed as if we were turning an important corner, I felt his presence even more. This was his legacy, after all.

It was a reminder, too, of how important all kinds of institutions are in the fight against AIDS. Not just governments but corporations, religious groups, charities. How much good they can do, how many resources they can amass, and how much influence they can impart. It was a reminder of possibility – the possibility that we *could* end AIDS forever if we tried.

Maybe that's why the *New York Times* article I read one morning that May of 2003 felt like such a punch to the gut. It opened like this:

> A division of the pharmaceutical company Bayer sold millions of dollars of blood-clotting medicine for hemophiliacs – medicine that carried a high risk of transmitting AIDS – to Asia and Latin America in the mid-1980s while selling a new, safer product in the West, according to documents obtained by the *New York Times*.[1]

The medicine the article was referencing was factor VIII, the same medicine that had caused Ryan to contract HIV. In the early 1980s, the evidence was overwhelming that factor VIII was dangerous in its current form. And so Bayer, the drug's manufacturer, introduced a safer version in 1984.

According to the *Times*, the company had a large surplus of the old, HIV-tainted factor VIII, and they weren't about to throw it away. That would waste costs. So instead, they sold it. Abroad.

Bayer claimed this wasn't their fault. Customers still wanted the old stuff, as they doubted the new drug's effectiveness, so Bayer gave it to them. Some countries, they said, were slow to approve the new drug. There was also a shortage of plasma for the new medicine.

They were simply meeting demand, they claimed. When doctors in Hong Kong, who had become worried about the growing number of haemophiliac patients with HIV, asked for the new factor VIII, Bayer urged them to use up their existing stocks of the old, infected treatment first. And that's not all. The company kept manufacturing the old product as well, even *after* they knew that each batch had the potential to transmit HIV.

As the *Times* reported, the company already had a lot of fixed-price contracts in place, so they were going to get paid the same amount whether they sold the new drug or the old one. And the old one was cheaper to make.

'These are the most incriminating internal pharmaceutical industry documents I have ever seen,' Dr Sidney M. Wolfe, director of the Public Citizen Health Research Group, told the *Times*. Indeed, in February 1985, a full year after the newer, safer product had been introduced, an internal company task force asked, quite simply, 'Can we in good faith continue to ship [potentially tainted] products to Japan?' They couldn't – not in good faith, not with a clear conscience. But they did.

It's impossible to know how many people died because of Bayer's actions. What we do know is that the company exported more than 100,000 vials of potentially tainted factor VIII after they had already begun selling the safer product elsewhere. We know those transactions were worth $4 million – about $8 million in today's dollars.

While Bayer still insists on its innocence in the matter, it was only recently discovered in 2011 that the company reached a settlement – without any admission of liability – in the protracted legal battle that resulted from its reprehensible actions. The exact details of the settlement have not been disclosed, but according to one source, Bayer agreed to pay $50 million in restitution.[2]

Bayer said in the *Times* that Cutter (the division of the company that sold factor VIII) had behaved 'responsibly, ethically and humanely' in continuing to sell the original drug overseas. But as far as I am concerned, it was greed – this was business, after all, and business is about money, not lives. We all know the power of greed. But this story is a stark reminder of the terribly evil decisions people make in the name of profits. It is a story we should never, ever forget.

As I read the details in that article, I thought of Ryan and ached for the unnamed thousands who had died just like he did. Ryan, like so many of my friends, contracted the disease too soon, before we had any real treatment, before we knew what was causing it and how to prevent it. But how many people must there have been, in Hong Kong, in Taiwan, in Argentina, and elsewhere, who didn't need to contract the disease at all? Who didn't need to die?

A year earlier, I had told the congressional committee, 'The drug companies are the only organisations in the world whose resources can rival those of rich governments in battling the disease.' But, I also told Congress, 'they have broken a public trust. They can't expect to keep pulling in profits, have their research subsidised, and then go missing in the midst of a worldwide health emergency. They can't keep telling us they're in the business of saving lives, if they always put business *ahead* of saving lives. We need them – and everyone – as partners.'

What I was referencing in my testimony was not the evil actions of the pharmaceutical industry; it was the evil of *inaction*.

As I wrote earlier, there have been extraordinary advances in AIDS treatments over the last thirty years, a true testament to the incredible brilliance of researchers and scientists who dedicated themselves to ending the disease. A lot of those scientists are employed by drug companies. A lot of them aren't.

What drug companies will tell you is that pharmaceutical development doesn't just happen. It requires big investments, sometimes hundreds of millions of dollars; it requires years of testing, sometimes more than a decade, through several rigorous phases. If things don't work out, if the drug fails, the companies are on the hook for the entire investment. And if they do work, companies need to make back the money they invested – plus a reasonable profit – when their new drug is sold.

This is just how it works, they'll tell you, and it's why, as sorry as they may be about it, the AIDS drugs on the market are very expensive – prohibitively so for the vast majority of people in the world living with the disease. There is just no other way around it.

But this is only half true. Maybe less than half.

It is incredibly rare for pharmaceutical companies to be working on the kind of research they are describing as so expensive without help – a lot of help – from taxpayers. Drug companies aren't the only ones investing in research. The biggest cost they face is shared. Much of the basic, critical research is funded by public or non-profit entities. This research doesn't even make it to the drug company until a big breakthrough has been made. And even then, the drug companies get funding to turn the breakthroughs into something they can sell.

AmfAR, for example, has invested more than $340 million and issued grants to more than 2,000 research teams. The work they've funded is largely responsible for the development of all kinds of HIV treatments.

They funded the research that showed how antiretro-virals could block mother-to-infant transmission of the disease. Their grants helped improve diagnostic and monitoring capabilities, and research they've enabled has helped us to understand the virus better. Currently amfAR is funding HIV vaccine research.

And that's just one non-profit organisation. The U.S. government and the international community have spent billions of dollars on AIDS research to date. So the drug companies are not, as they claim, doing this work on their own. And yet they charge prices as though they were. No wonder they are among the most profit-able companies in the world.

It's worth remembering that it was the CDC, not a drug company, that first warned the world about the HIV virus and first identified the ways in which it was transmitted. It was a doctor working at a French non-profit institute, not a drug company, who isolated the virus. It was the government-funded U.S. National Institutes of Health, not a drug company, that spear-headed the initial research into the disease. It was amfAR that sponsored the research into the protease inhibitors that worked as second-line treatments. And in 1996, it was a researcher named David Ho, director not of a private drug lab but of the non-profit Aaron Diamond AIDS Research Center in New York City, who discovered the so-called AIDS cocktail of life-saving medicine, using those same protease inhibitors investigated by amfAR, that would revolutionise treatment for millions of people living with HIV/AIDS.

I don't write this to suggest that the drug companies have no role. They play a crucial one. But I have strong objections to the story they prefer telling and the consequences of it. The distance we have come with AIDS treatment is one of the greatest collective achievements of humankind. It is not, as they would have you believe, a product entirely of the pharmaceutical industry's own work.

The truth is, the drug companies can afford to sell AIDS medication for less – a lot less – and still make a fine profit. They have the power to act, to step up, and to become the boldest leaders of all in the fight to end the disease. I'm not saying that drug companies shouldn't earn a profit. They wouldn't exist if they couldn't make money, and we very much need them to exist. The question is, does their profit on life-saving drugs have to be so high that it prevents them from saving lives as intended?

Let me put it this way. Pretend for a moment that you are a multibillion-dollar, multinational drug company. If you found out that you could save millions of lives and make a profit while doing it but that your profit margin would be just slightly less than it is now, would you do it?

How about if I sweeten the deal? What if you had to charge a lot less for your AIDS medicine in the developing world, but in exchange for doing so, you could get access to millions of new customers? What if your per-pill profits were smaller, but in the aggregate, you could make more money than you do now because suddenly you were flush with new orders? And what if I told you that those millions of customers whose lives you were saving were going to need to take the pills you produce every single day for the rest of their lives?

In other words, what if I told you I could get you millions of lifelong customers you would otherwise have no access to, and profits for as long as AIDS exists? And all you have to do is lower the price.

Who *wouldn't* take that deal?

This isn't a hypothetical scenario. This was an actual deal offered to the major brand-name drug companies by the William J. Clinton Foundation a number of years ago. A deal they outright rejected.

In 2002, former president Bill Clinton's foundation began to take on the issue of AIDS. President Clinton has often said that he regrets not doing far more to fight AIDS when he was in the White House. I regret that he didn't do more as well. But, since he left office, the work of his foundation has been game changing.

The Clinton Foundation started in the Bahamas, where they discovered that the government was paying about $3,600 a year per person for generic AIDS drugs, instead of the list price of $500. 'How could this be?' they asked. Upon investigating, the Clinton Foundation discovered that middlemen were jacking up the prices. So they called up the generic manufacturer and made a deal that cut out these middlemen and made the drugs a whole lot cheaper for the Bahamian government to buy.[3]

That episode sparked the interest of the former president and his staff. Were AIDS drugs more expensive than they had to be? Could something be done about that?

President Clinton put together a small team of management consultants who figured out a couple of important things: First, they concluded that they could streamline the drug companies' operations, making it cheaper to produce the drugs. Then they figured out they could do the same thing for every company along the supply chain. Make everything run faster, better, more efficiently, and you make everything cheaper.

But this was just the start. Next, their plan was to get the drug companies to produce at a much greater scale, which would make each individual pill far less expensive to manufacture. It's like when you go to the grocery store: you can buy one soda for $1 or a twelve-pack for $6, which is just $0.50 per soda. Half the price. Buy a twenty-four-pack for $8, and now it's just $0.34 a soda. Imagine how cheap it would get if, instead of buying twenty-four sodas, you were buying twenty-four thousand. The price per soda would drop to pennies.

So the idea was simple enough: if the drug manu-facturers produced a lot more drugs, the drugs them-selves would be a whole lot cheaper to make and thus to sell. That would mean, with the same government expenditure, far more drugs could be purchased and many more lives could be saved.

The problem was that no drug company was going to make more drugs if it couldn't be sure it would have customers to buy them. At the time, the Clinton Foundation estimated there were only about 70,000 people receiving treatment in the developing world. But there were millions who needed it.[4]

That's where the foundation stepped in. First, they went to governments in Africa and the Caribbean and made a basic pitch: If we can get you cheap AIDS drugs, will you commit to buying a lot of them? Then they went to the drug companies and made the reverse pitch: If we can get you 2 million customers in the developing world, help you make your operation and supply chain a lot more efficient, and guarantee you a profit, will you sell your drugs for a lot less than you do now?

The governments said yes. But the brand-name drug companies balked. They didn't want any part of it.

I'm not sure what President Clinton said in those meetings. He's one of the most persuasive men on earth, that much is well known. And this was, after all, a great deal. The drug companies were going to make good money, and they were going to make it from selling drugs to a huge population of customers they didn't have access to. And that's just the business piece of it – countless lives would be saved as well. But the companies turned down the offer. Somehow they had found a way to reject a deal that would have made them more money and made a real impact in the fight against AIDS at the same time.

The good news is that Bill Clinton is not easily dissuaded. If the brand-name manufacturers wouldn't step up to the plate, fine, he would take his offer elsewhere. His foundation approached generic manufacturers in India, South Africa, Thailand, and other countries, and asked if they were interested in the same deal. But there was a catch: if the generic companies manufactured the drugs, they'd be at risk of violating the patents of brand-name companies. He told them to go for it anyway. They'd have his full support. 'No company will live or die because of high price premiums for AIDS drugs in middle-income countries,' Clinton said in Thailand, 'but patients may.'[5]

The Clinton Foundation held up their end of the bargain. So did the generic drug manufacturers. And in May 2007, Clinton's foundation was able to announce an incredible deal. Prices would fall, on average, 25 per cent in low-income countries. They would fall, on average, 50 per cent in middle-income countries. And one-pill-a-day treatments would be made available for less than $1 for developing countries, which represented a 45 per cent discount in Africa. The deal, in total, would impact sixty-six nations all over the world. It was just this side of a miracle, and the major drug companies played no role in the equation whatsoever.

I've talked about the critical role of governments in fighting AIDS. I said that no institution was as capable of sweeping change. But governments alone will not solve this problem. Governments aren't the only institutions in our society. They're not the only players on the field. If we are going to rid the world of AIDS, we need a commitment from governments, yes, but we also need a commitment from many others. And we badly need a commitment from the drug makers.

The generic manufacturers have been quiet heroes in all of this. In fact, they supply some 80 to 90 per cent of all AIDS medicine worldwide. But the generics are tiny compared to the big guys. Globally, the brand-name companies bring in about eight times the market share of the generic companies. We need the big pharmaceuticals on board, too. I'm not asking them to become charities instead of companies. I'm not naive enough to think that would work, nor would it be wise. I'm asking only that they keep the faith with their missions a little better. If you can make money while saving lives, then more power to you. But if you choose to make even more money at the *expense* of people's lives, then you should be ashamed. The pharmaceutical companies have an obligation not just to their shareholders but also to the global public. If they ignore that obligation, the fight against AIDS will never be won.

This is a battle that requires as many reinforcements as possible, from every institution in our global society. And I should say that while governments are essential, and while drug companies are, too, they're not the only ones. We need other corporations, as many as are able to lend a hand. You'd be amazed what an effect they can have.

I remember back in 1987 when General Motors was one of the first major businesses outside Hollywood to launch an AIDS prevention and education programme for its employees. At the time they employed 519,000 workers. That's a lot of people who learned the details of the disease because executives at the company decided that AIDS mattered. And the fact that GM was willing to take this step, I'm sure, played a big role in other companies getting on board, too.

Or take a more contemporary example: Walgreens, America's largest drugstore chain, has designated more than five hundred of its pharmacies as 'HIV Centers of Excellence' in communities heavily affected by HIV/AIDS. These stores are staffed with specially trained pharmacists. Their shelves are fully stocked with anti-retrovirals, and many of these stores carry female condoms, which can be very hard to find. The pharmacists call their patients frequently. They work with drug companies to get medicine donated to patients who can't afford to pay. They even help those who are suffering through related crises – addiction, for example – to seek help or treatment.

This is how you make a difference. And, by the way, this is how you can make money while doing so. Walgreens is contributing to the fight against AIDS, of course, but I imagine they're also turning a profit by filling prescriptions and obtaining new customers. That's just fine by me. There's nothing wrong with doing good and doing well at the same time, as they say.

There are countless other ways corporations can have an impact. For example, our foundation partnered with the Kaiser Family Foundation and the Black AIDS Institute on Greater Than AIDS, a wonderful initiative among public and private sector partners that aims to educate and mobilise those most affected by the AIDS epidemic in America. As part of this effort, major media companies and other corporate allies are working alongside health departments and AIDS service and community-based organisations to increase the knowledge and understanding of HIV/AIDS and to confront the stigma surrounding the disease.

There are scores of corporations that have been essential to the fight, even if they aren't on the front lines themselves. Our foundation has received millions of dollars from hundreds of corporate donors over the last twenty years. There is an enormous amount of money pumping through the corporate world, and there are good-hearted people at these companies. I know this firsthand. Our goal should be to channel some of these resources and the efforts of corporate executives into the fight against AIDS.

In fact, every institution of influence, every institution with resources, must step up if we are to win this battle.

We can't do it alone. We can't do it with only some. We need everyone, from the boardrooms to the front lines. We need them all – governments, corporations, and, yes, even religious institutions. *Especially* religious institutions.

In the summer of 2010, the German journalist Peter Seewald sat down with Pope Benedict XVI over several days for an interview he planned to turn into a book. They spoke about a number of issues, but the one that caught the most public attention was the conversation they had about AIDS.

Seewald asked the pope about the church's efforts to fight AIDS, especially in light of its strict opposition to contraception. 'Critics,' Seewald said bluntly, 'object that it is madness to forbid a high-risk population to use condoms.' Pope Benedict gave a lengthy response. At the end of it, he seemed to do what AIDS advocates had demanded for as long as the disease has been known; he seemed to reverse the church's position on condoms:

> There may be a basis in the case of some individuals, as perhaps when a male prostitute uses a condom, where this can be a first step in the direction of a moralization, a first assumption of responsibility, on the way toward recovering an awareness that not everything is allowed and that one cannot do whatever one wants.[6]

Seewald was surprised by the pope's reply. 'Are you saying, then,' he asked, 'that the Catholic Church is actually not opposed in principle to the use of condoms?' Again, an astounding reversal from the pope:

> She of course does not regard it as a real or moral solution, but, in this or that case, there can be nonetheless, in the intention of reducing the risk of infection, a first step in a movement toward a different way, a more human way, of living sexuality.[7]

Now, if you're like me, you could read the pope's words a dozen times and still wonder what in God's name (literally) he is talking about. But when reports of these quotes broke, there was a sense of utter elation. It turns out that even these contorted statements were a radical departure from the church's deeply held, long-time position against condoms.

In the fight against AIDS, I'm sorry to say, there have been few institutions more destructive than the Catholic Church itself. And to a large degree this has been due to the church's stance on condoms. In the late 1960s, Pope Paul VI sent a papal letter to all the bishops of the church, laying out his – and their – official position. He outright rejected the use of contraception of any kind, in any circumstance, saying it was 'to be absolutely excluded as lawful means of regulating the number of children."[8]

The impact of that decree was felt worldwide long before the AIDS crisis emerged. But in the '80s and '90s, when it became clear that there was a deadly sexually transmitted disease ravaging populations, that there was no cure for it, and that the only method to prevent transmission was the use of condoms, the church's position became all the more untenable. It wasn't just leading to unwanted pregnancies; it was leading to death – by the millions.

Sadly, Pope John Paul II was horrifically rigid. Just a few months after Ryan White died, the pope travelled to Africa, where he emphasised, even while talking about the need to combat AIDS, that contraception was a sin. It is not at all an exaggeration to say that his words were deadly.[9] I hold him personally responsible for all those who died as a result of heeding his advice, or who couldn't access condoms due to his ill-founded and immoral decree. I've said before that his words resulted in genocide, and I stand by that statement. For as much love and adoration as there is in the world for Pope John Paul II, I will never forgive him for this.

What's worse, if you can imagine anything worse, the church actively *misinformed* its worshippers. It's one thing, I suppose, to tell people that the use of condoms is a sin. It is entirely another to tell them that condoms do not work at all. And yet that's exactly what happened. As *The Guardian* reported in 2003, 'The Catholic Church is telling people in countries stricken with AIDS not to use condoms because they have tiny holes in them through which HIV can pass.'[10]

This, of course, is categorically untrue. The correct use of condoms reduces the risk of HIV transmission by 90 per cent. But that didn't stop the church from preaching otherwise. It didn't stop Pope Benedict XVI, in 2009, from saying in Africa that the use of condoms actually makes the problem of HIV worse.[11] Nor did it stop the church from lobbying for a law in El Salvador that required condoms to carry a false warning label that said they don't protect against HIV.[12]

It's essential to note here that not everyone in the Catholic Church agrees with this position and that countless Catholics, especially nuns and priests who minister to people living with HIV/AIDS, have chosen to reject the church's dogma. They encourage the people they work with to use condoms. They find the church position impossible to square with the death and suffering it has unleashed.

I've met a lot of these dedicated and faithful Catholics. Our foundation has worked with them in many different countries. To spend any time with these caring priests and nuns is to know that *they* are the real church. They are the people truly obeying and representing the teachings of Christ. I remember Nicholas Kristof of the *New York Times* recounting a story of a priest in Brazil, who told him, 'If I were pope, I would start a condom factory right in the Vatican. What's the point of sending food and medicine when we let people get infected with AIDS and die?'[13]

Given this sordid history, all the unnecessary suffering and death, you can understand how important it was to have Pope Benedict shift the church's position, if only slightly. I have to give him credit for that, even as I reject what he's said about condoms making the AIDS crisis worse. He hasn't gone as far as I want him to, or as far as we need him to, and his position seems contradictory at best. But this fiercely conservative pope has taken a first step toward a change in the church's position on condoms – a step few thought he would ever take, on a road that could lead, if the Vatican chooses, toward the eradication of AIDS.

If we can't do it without government on our side, or drug companies on our side, or corporations on our side, we certainly can't do it without religious institutions on our side. Their power is too great, their influence too far-reaching, for us to succeed with them as our adversaries. And so we need them to stand with us in the fight against AIDS. Yes, that means outreach and treatment and support – which, in fairness, the Catholic Church does quite a bit of. But it means more than that. It means encouraging prevention based on logic and science. It means rejecting stigma instead of re-inforcing it. It means ending, once and for all, the misinformation campaign that is killing people all over the world.

This is especially true for the Catholic Church, both because of its history and because of its extraordinary reach with some 1 billion faithful. But it is crucial for all religions, all houses of worship, no matter how big or small, in all nations. There is no excuse for furthering pain and injustice in the name of any god. As I've said, I am not a religious man. But I know there is no god, not in any religion, who believes we should turn our backs on the sick. No god could possibly condone inaction and misinformation that result in death. No loving god could possibly embrace those consequences.

These, as I see it, are the major institutions that matter most and that have the most responsibility to act. Governments. Corporations. Religious organisations. They each have the power to respond to the AIDS crisis in different ways. They each have the ability to do extraordinary good and terrible harm, and they all have that choice to make for themselves.

But even if they act responsibly, even if they join together in common cause to end this disease, they still cannot do it *entirely* alone. There are roles they can't – or, at least, won't – ever take on. And that leaves holes in the strategy, gaps that can be filled only by non-profit organisations working within civil society.

Think about it. President Clinton was able to cut the price of AIDS drugs by doing something with his foundation that he never could have done from the White House: encouraging other nations to violate international patents. That's an example of a big non-profit organisation doing big things. But there are small organisations, too, foundations not run by ex-presidents, non-profits working on the front lines, doing work you won't ever see governments do.

For instance, EJAF funds a fantastic Washington, DC-based organisation called HIPS, which stands for 'Helping Individual Prostitutes Survive.' They're focused entirely on sex workers living with HIV or at risk of contracting it. That's a marginalised, stigmatised population that we have to assist if we're going to end the disease, but it's one the American government won't be supporting anytime soon, I can assure you.

Without non-profits, critical work like this would go undone. Charitable organisations have a tremendous role to play in fighting AIDS and a tremendous responsibility as well, just like every other institution I've discussed here. Because the work of non-profits is essential, the way they undergo their work is essential, too. Non-profits must act appropriately and with the same accountability that we demand of governments and corporations and religious institutions.

Whether you're operating a grant-making foundation like EJAF, or a small on-the-ground organisation like the many we fund, the strength of the operation determines the reach of its impact. And that matters a great deal. If we're going to end this disease, the impact of non-profits must reach as far as possible. Resources are so precious that we can't be wasteful; otherwise, we're harming the cause.

There are a lot of wonderful people who want to do important work. They have what they believe is a unique idea, and they decide to start a non-profit. But what some fail to do before they start, or even after, is to determine whether another organisation is already doing what they've set out to undertake. Sometimes non-profits re-invent the wheel without realising it. Other times they figure out that they're duplicating another organisation's effort, but they convince themselves that they can do it better anyway. Sometimes they're right, sometimes that works out. But too often it doesn't, and scarce funds are wasted.

If you're going to start your own organisation, more power to you. I think it's fantastic, and for me, it's been a life-changing experience. But it's essential that new organisations fill a need that isn't already being met. Otherwise it's a waste of that organisation's time and its donors' money. Non-profit organisations that work together on a particular issue need to see themselves as part of a single strategic team, not as isolated players.

This was the core of EJAF's operating philosophy in the early 1990s, and it remains so today. We figured the thing we could do better than others was raise money. But rather than trying to determine the best way to use the money we raised (which would have itself cost a lot of money), EJAF-U.S. found an organisation that had figured out how to do that already – the National Community AIDS Partnership. Instead of hiring teams of people to go out on the front lines, we identified organisations that were already on the ground doing the work, and we made sure they had funding to be successful.

Indeed, at the UK arm of my foundation alone, through strategic partnerships we've leveraged an additional $350 million on top of the funds that have been raised directly by EJAF. In the United States, we've leveraged another $127 million. Simply by working with other organisations to fight AIDS in a coordinated and united way, we've greatly increased our direct impact.

This idea of leverage must be paramount for non-profits, most of which have very limited resources. Finding opportunities to maximise those resources through programming or fund-raising partnerships is essential. It's like the old saying: 'The whole is greater than the sum of its parts.' In my experience, any achievements made in charitable work are *collective* achievements. Leveraging partnerships is not only a very good idea; it is an absolute necessity.

Ultimately, perhaps more than anything else, non-profits need credibility to succeed. And that credibility comes not just from success in the field but also from proof that the headquarters are being run as efficiently as possible. It matters to donors, who may choose to write a large cheque or withhold a large cheque, depending on how the operation is being handled. When you lose credibility on how you run your organisation, you lose donations. And when you lose donations, you lose the ability to meet your mission.

That's why I'm most proud of the fact that EJAF has operated with relentless efficiency from day one. Ever since the years when we were scraping by with a makeshift office in John Scott's kitchen, we have continued to keep our overhead costs as low as possible. As a result of the tight ship we run, EJAF has been awarded

Charity Navigator's highest four-star rating for seven years in a row. More important, our efficiency is why we've received such tremendous support from many wonderful individuals and corporate sponsors over the years. Our donors know that we take our work and their contributions seriously, and that their funds will be used wisely to achieve maximum impact.

So, you see, we all have a role to play. Governments, corporations, religious institutions, and civil society. We can't afford to have anyone on the sidelines. We are all responsible for ending AIDS, and we must all contribute to that worthy goal. But none of us can succeed alone. Beating this epidemic will require every major institution of modern life to fight together and find common cause despite vast differences. That is an incredibly daunting task, uniting the world in this way. But I believe it *can* be done.

If we work together, and with compassion at the centre of our efforts, it really is possible to end AIDS.

10

Ending AIDS Forever

You might think that I'm naive, plain and simple. Just another celebrity with a foundation, another rock star who thinks he has the answer to the world's ills. AIDS is a deadly disease, not something we can wish away with sappy sentiments and positive thinking. This is the real world, and it's not always a nice one. There is so much fighting, so much hate. How could *love* be the cure for anything at all?

When it comes to AIDS, however, love *is* the cure. Indeed, as of this moment, and for the foreseeable future, it is the *only* cure.

AIDS isn't like other diseases. It's special, you could say. Consider the difference between AIDS and cancer. If you were able to treat everyone with cancer on the planet, if you could give everyone the best, most cutting-edge treatment possible, other people would still get cancer. And, sadly, a lot of those who received treatment would still die.

The same goes for other diseases among the top killers worldwide, such as heart disease, or stroke, or diabetes. Existing science alone can't yet abolish these afflictions. We don't yet know how to fully treat or fully prevent these epidemics. We will need further medical advances to accomplish that.

But, at this point, if all AIDS research were to suddenly stop, if we were never to make another discovery in our understanding of the HIV virus, we could still beat it. We could save the life of nearly *every* HIV-positive person and prevent *all* future infections. We could end AIDS. And that is an *amazing* fact. It's a fact that makes AIDS rather unique among the world's deadliest pandemics.

Right now, while we don't yet have a cure for AIDS, we do have the next best thing: medicine that can return dying AIDS patients to near perfect health and give them very long lives. There can sometimes be unpleasant side-effects of the medication, of course, as with many drugs. And some people, like my friend Eli, can still lose their lives to complications, despite receiving the very best medical treatment.

But today's treatments are overwhelmingly life-saving, and that's the bottom line. HIV is no longer a death sentence. With treatment, HIV morphs from a lethal virus into a chronic condition that can be managed.

With treatment, almost every single HIV-positive person can live happily, comfortably, productively, and – to echo my friend Ryan's only wish – *normally*. Today, you can be HIV-positive and lead a very normal life indeed.

What's more, if we made treatment universal, over time, we could end the AIDS epidemic *forever*.

Let me explain.

In 2011, researchers funded by the U.S. government made a miraculous discovery: people living with HIV who receive treatment are up to *96 per cent less likely* to pass on the virus to a sexual partner. In other words, current treatments are so effective that they reduce the presence of the HIV virus in an infected person's body to almost nil. The chance of infecting others plummets as a result. That means *treatment is also prevention*. And therefore if we treat everyone, we can drastically reduce the spread of HIV. By giving medication to every single person living with HIV/AIDS in the world today – or even *almost* everyone – we can prevent tens of millions of future infections. We would save millions of lives of those already infected, yes, but we would also begin to end this disease by stopping it from spreading.

At the same time, we must double-down on other highly effective and proven preventive measures. Free condoms, sex education, and needle exchange programmes are essential components of any effort to end AIDS.

Ideally, we would provide these to marginalised and high-risk populations such as sex workers, injection drug users, and men who have sex with men. Also, it turns out that heterosexual men who are circumcised are about 60 per cent less likely to pass HIV to a sexual partner, and therefore many AIDS advocates suggest voluntary male circumcision as a very important tool to stop the spread of HIV. Finally, to keep AIDS on the run, we must also ensure that all those who receive medication stay on it for the rest of their lives. That's because of the way our current treatments work. If people with HIV stop taking their medicine, the virus comes roaring back. Even worse, it can come back stronger, more virulent, and potentially resistant to today's treatments. If many HIV-positive people were to stop taking their medicine all at once, it could trigger a new AIDS epidemic, one that we might not be able to treat or prevent.

Consider, then, where we are today in the treatment and prevention of HIV/AIDS. We have amazing drugs that can hold the virus at bay indefinitely and all but stop it from spreading. We have prevention methods that can further eliminate any chance of transmitting the virus. What this means is that we don't need to wait for a vaccine for HIV, though I desperately hope we will find one soon. What we need to end AIDS *right now* is the compassion, the empathy, the commitment, and, yes, the love to make sure that everyone who is HIV-positive has access to existing treatments and established prevention methods.

You can't say that about cancer or heart disease or practically any other epidemic. But because of the efforts of scientists and doctors and researchers all over the world, you *can* say that about AIDS. If we can find the love as a global community to agree that every life has equal value, if we can summon the compassion to provide treatment and prevention for everyone living with HIV – and I mean *everyone*, no matter who they are, where they live, or how rich or poor they may be – we can end AIDS forever. We can prevent 34 million people from dying and tens of millions more from getting sick in the first place, and we can contain the virus itself among those already infected. Over time, as HIV-positive people would live normal lives and die normal deaths, new infections would plummet, and the HIV virus would simply cease to exist. The AIDS epidemic would be over.

Can you imagine that? *An AIDS-free world.* The very thought makes my heart leap. And it's entirely within our grasp. This isn't a fairy tale; it's really, truly possible. We can cure this disease without a cure. We can end AIDS with love.

That is why the reality of AIDS treatment and prevention today is so incredibly tragic. For all the progress being made in expanding HIV treatment around the world, it is still the case that not even *half* of the 14.2 million people in low- and middle-income countries in need of antiretroviral therapy received it in 2010. That means there is still a lot of work to be done. What's more, we aren't widely implementing the prevention efforts that are proven to be effective. In some places, we are not even implementing them at all.

You might think this is because it's simply too expensive to provide treatment and prevention to all who need it. After all, so much in our world comes down to dollars and cents. Surely it must cost a fortune to purchase medicine for tens of millions of people with HIV and, in so doing, begin to end the epidemic. If such a thing were possible, if such a thing were *affordable*, we would have done it already, you might reasonably conclude. Money must be why humanity has not taken the necessary steps to end AIDS.

I wish that were true. I wish it were a matter of resources alone. But it isn't. It's a matter of compassion. It all comes down to love.

In 2011, experts at UNAIDS; the Global Fund to Fight AIDS, Tuberculosis, and Malaria; PEPFAR; the Gates Foundation; the World bank; and the World

Health Organization, among others, conducted an exhaustive joint study.[1] They modelled a way to use all existing treatments and proven prevention methods to end AIDS. Then they tallied the cost and determined how resources would need to be spent over time. What they concluded is astonishing.

According to UNAIDS, in 2010 some $15 billion was available worldwide to fight AIDS in the developing world.[2] The consortium of experts determined that it would take only an additional $5 to $7 billion per year to go from treatment and prevention for *some*, to treatment and prevention for *all who need it*. This additional spending would, the experts say, prevent 12.2 million new infections and save 7.4 million lives between 2011 and 2020 alone.

Initially, funding would ramp up, but then it would steadily decline. Worldwide spending would need to rise from $16.6 billion in 2011 to $22 billion per year in 2015, and from that point it would drop to $19.8 billion in 2020. After 2020, the cost of a worldwide campaign to end AIDS would continue to decline precipitously, because far fewer people would become newly infected and the cost of treatment would drop for those already living with HIV.

And there you have it. We know how to end AIDS, and we know what it would cost: an additional $5 to

$7 billion each year from now until 2020, and not very much more than we're spending today beyond that.

At first, this sounds like quite a lot of money. In the hands of an individual, it would be an incredible windfall. If you had several billion dollars, you'd be one of the richest people on earth. But when you put several billion dollars in the context of other spending, you quickly realise that it's not very much money at all. In fact, it's a tiny, almost meaningless sum in the grand scheme of things.

Consider that in 2010, Americans alone spent $11 billion on vitamins, $16.9 billion on chocolate, and $18.7 billion on pet food. A handful of Wall Street banks paid out $20.8 billion in bonuses to employees and executives that same year. More recently Apple, Inc., made profits of $13 billion in the first quarter of 2012 alone. In fact, at the beginning of 2012, Apple had cash reserves of $96.7 billion. That's right; a single corporation has, sitting in its bank account, far more than the additional funds we would need to finance a global campaign to end the AIDS epidemic.

I'm not suggesting that Americans should starve their pets or that Apple should use iPhone profits to fight AIDS. My point is simply this: the several billion dollars in additional spending needed to end AIDS is a pittance when compared to even minute snapshots of global commerce. And for governments – especially in Western countries, developed economies, and large developing countries – several billion dollars a year is the practical equivalent of the change in your pocket.

I mean that quite literally. Take the United States, for instance, the world's richest nation, with the largest economy. The budget of the American government in 2011 was $3.7 *trillion*. This is an incomprehensibly large figure. For reference, a billion is to a trillion dollars what $1 is to $1,000. If you had $3,700 in your current account, would you not part with an extra $5 to $7 to save millions upon millions of lives?

I should say here that the U.S. government has already pledged $48 billion to PEPFAR from 2009 to 2013 to fight AIDS, tuberculosis, and malaria in the developing world. And in 2010, the Kaiser Family Foundation estimated that the United States provided 54.2 per cent of all international AIDS assistance.[3] The American people and their government are doing more than any other nation to fight this disease, and Americans should be very proud of this fact. Indeed, they should be celebrated for it. But imagine, with another $5 to $7 billion per year – a rounding error in the federal budget – the United States could *single-handedly* end AIDS. For a small fraction of what was spent on the war in Iraq, America would forever be heralded as the country that won the war against AIDS. And yet this need not be an American burden to bear. Governments of the world could easily commit the necessary funds to end AIDS. The cost would be a single drop in the vast ocean of worldwide government spending. The money would not even be missed.

I don't mean to suggest that money is the *only* thing we need to end AIDS. It is absolutely necessary, but not by any means sufficient. In addition to greater resources, we need greater understanding, and that is where you, my dear reader, come in.

HIV/AIDS is a disease that not only attacks the human immune system; it attacks the human social system. It infects our civic institutions with fear, our communities with hate, our corporations with greed, our churches and synagogues and mosques with loathing. There is no medicine, no creation of science, that will inoculate us from these social afflictions. And that is why the cure for AIDS is a matter of changing hearts and educating minds.

To end AIDS, we need countries like Uganda to change their laws so we can reach gay people in need of help. We need the Catholic Church to stop telling its members that condoms are sinful, and even worse that they do not work. We need pharmaceutical companies to give up some profits in the name of humanity. We need charitable organisations to keep up the amazing work they are doing, marching forward with a vengeance and moving the front lines of our fight against AIDS.

But these institutions aren't nameless, faceless monoliths. They start with individuals, and they are guided by individuals. Whether they do good or ill is up to individual choice. And while the disease is bigger than any one of us, the cure requires something from each of us.

It requires us to talk to our partners, to practise safe sex, and to get tested, and we must encourage friends and loved ones to do the same. It requires us to stand up for those living with HIV/AIDS and those most at risk of becoming infected. It requires us to educate ourselves about what governments and religious organisations are doing – and not doing – in our names. It requires us to embrace all those who need and deserve our compassion.

In other words, ending AIDS requires love, and lots of it. And the best way to engender love is to foster dialogue. We can only love one another if we understand one another. That is why I have written this book. And I hope that you will talk about what you have read here with others. When AIDS is an uncomfortable and untouchable subject, the disease spreads. But when we bring it to the fore, when we aren't afraid to confront it, information spreads. Compassion spreads. The cure spreads.

Please, help me spread the cure.

Ending this disease is no longer a matter of money. And it is no longer a matter of technology. It is a matter of finding the will to do what is necessary to save countless lives and beat this terrible pandemic. It's a matter of fighting stigma and politics, intolerance and indifference. The question is not whether we *can* do it, or whether we can *afford* to do it. The question is whether we *care* enough to do it.

No one is blameless in this terrible equation of apathy. Including me. I am the first to stand up and say that I did not do enough. I did not care enough. But I have changed. And so can we all. So can our institutions. So can our communities. So can our global society. I believe that with every fibre of my being. If I didn't believe it, I wouldn't have written this book. If I didn't believe it, I would have simply given up. But I won't give up, I never will, because I have seen the power of compassion. I won't give up, because I believe in love.

In 2009, David and I visited an AIDS orphanage in Donetsk, Ukraine. It was a familiar scene to me, I'm sad to say. Dozens of children, perhaps even a hundred, many of whom were HIV-positive, many of whom were only infants and toddlers, living in dorm-like conditions and being looked after by a wonderful but terribly under-resourced staff.

A boy gravitated toward me. He was eighteen months old, and his name was Lev. In an instant, he stole my heart. I held Lev, and I was in love. I had always said I was too old, too selfish, too set in my ways to have children, even though David was keen for us to have a family one day. The truth is that I love children – David and I are godparents many times over. But with our hectic schedules, with my travelling on tour constantly, it didn't seem like it would ever work out for us to have a child of our own.

All that changed the minute Lev's eyes met mine. David and I tried to adopt Lev. We were heart-broken that Ukraine's draconian laws prevented us from doing so without waiting several years, during which time Lev would have to remain in the orphanage. I couldn't stomach that, so instead Lev and his brother went to live with their grandmother.

It was then that David and I decided to have a child. Lev had sent us a message we could not ignore. Our son, Zachary, was born on Christmas Day in 2010.

Zachary is the light of our lives. Already he has taught me so much about life, and so much about love. In a very real way, the stories I've told here – the lessons they've taught me – are how I came to be blessed with my beautiful son.

I would not have Zachary but for the strangers who demonstrated such care and compassion for me at the lowest moments of my life. I would not have Zachary but for my friendship with Ryan White. I would not have Zachary but for my decision twenty years ago to make it up to Ryan and those I had let down because of my addictions and indifference. I would not have Zachary but for the creation of EJAF. I would not have Zachary but for my visit with David to the AIDS orphanage in Donetsk.

I would not have Zachary but for love.

It comes down to a simple equation, really. If you give love out, you get love back. If you take nothing else from the stories I've told here, please take that lesson to heart. It's the only thing that matters. It's why we need a global movement for love, and not just when it comes to AIDS. We need to love the poor, we need to love the sick, and we need to love those who we perceive as different. If love drives our actions, we can end AIDS. If love drives our actions, we can build a better world.

Every day, I watch Zachary learn a little more about life. Everything to him is fresh, everything is new. There is no hate in his heart, only wonder. We all came into the world that way. Our attitudes are learned from others. Our perspectives are shaped by experience. Zachary is learning from David and from me. Other children are learning from their families, from their communities, from the world around them and how they are treated by it. We can teach love as easily as we can teach hate.

Let us teach Zachary and his generation the power of love. Let us do so by ending AIDS.

Acknowledgements

First and foremost, I would like to thank my partner in all things, including this book, David Furnish. As chairman of the Elton John AIDS Foundation, David plays an instrumental role in the work you have read about here. EJAF is our joint passion, and I couldn't have written this book without his love, inspiration, guidance, and significant effort.

Scott Campbell, the executive director of EJAF-U.S., and Anne Aslett, the executive director of EJAF-UK, are, along with David, the reason my foundation has had such an incredible impact in recent years. Scott and Anne are more than trusted advisers and dedicated professionals. They are also very dear friends, and I thank them both for making this book possible and for their tireless work on behalf of EJAF.

I would also like to thank EJAF's staff in London and New York for continually achieving results far beyond their small numbers. I am grateful each and every day for their innumerable contributions to the fight against AIDS. They are the authors of this book as much as I am.

EJAF's outsize impact is due not only to its dedicated leadership and staff but also to its brilliant board of directors, which comprises many old friends who are deeply and personally dedicated to our mission and our work. EJAF is profoundly lucky to draw on their wisdom, passion, and ingenuity. In addition, we could not function – indeed we would not exist – without the extraordinary generosity of our donors and sponsors. So many supporters have been on the journey with us and shared our vision for years and years. Time and again, they came through when it was most needed. It's no exaggeration to say that their generosity has saved and transformed countless lives.

I've told many stories in this book of people from around the world – people living with AIDS; people on the front lines of the fight against the epidemic; people who are fighting for their lives, for the lives of others, and for a more just society. These people are real-life heroes. They are my heroes. Their struggles and their resilience have inspired me deeply. I wrote this book because I wanted the world to know their stories, and I thank them all for the opportunity to share something of their lives – and, I hope, to improve the lives of many others in so doing.

While I have been intimately involved in the fight against AIDS for twenty years, I am no expert on the history or science of the HIV/AIDS epidemic. That's why I have drawn on the work of many gifted researchers, journalists, academics, and AIDS advocates throughout this book. We should all be grateful that they have dedicated their professional efforts to helping the world better understand this disease and spreading information that contributes so greatly to fighting it.

I was thrilled when Michael Pietsch decided to take on this project. He believed in the message of the book from day one, and I appreciate his many insights and contributions, as well as those of his terrific staff at Little, Brown.

Finally, I would like to thank Ben Yarrow, a long-time partner of EJAF on our strategic communications, for working with me on this book and helping me bring it to fruition. Ben and his outstanding team at West Wing Writers – Ryan Clancy, David Heifetz, Dylan Loewe, Brittney Moraski, and Sarada Peri – were wonderful collaborators, and I am very grateful to have had the benefit of their many talents.

Notes

CHAPTER 1: RYAN

1 Ryan White and Marie Cunningham, *Ryan White: My Own Story* (New York: Signet, 1992), 93, 134, 135.

2 Cory SerVaas, 'The Happier Days for Ryan White,' *Saturday Evening Post*, March 1, 1988.

CHAPTER 2: A DECADE OF LOSS

1 Avert, 'History of AIDS up to 1986,' accessed February 23, 2012, http://www.avert.org/aids-history-86.htm.

2 Lawrence K. Altman, 'Rare Cancer Seen in 41 Homosexuals,' *New York Times*, July 3, 1981, accessed February 14, 2012, http://www.nytimes.com/1981/07/03/us/rare-cancer-seen-in-41-homosexuals.html.

3 'Fear of AIDS Infects the Nation,' *U.S. News & World Report*, June 27, 1983.

4 Randy Shilts, *And the Band Played On: Politics, People, and the AIDS Epidemic*, 20th anniversary ed. (New York: St Martin's Griffin, 1988), 299.

5 John G. Roberts and Deborah K. Owen, 'Presidential Briefing Memo,' *Frontline*, accessed December 23, 2011,

http://www.pbs.org/wgbh/pages/frontline/aids/docs/robertsmemo.html.

6   Shilts, *And the Band*, 321.

7   Jack Friedman and David Van Biema, 'Breaking America's Heart,' *People* 28, no. 5 (1987), accessed December 15, 2011, http://www.people.com/people/archive/article/0,,20199548,00.html.

8   Shilts, *And the Band*, 321.

9   Ibid., 352–53.

10 Ibid., 324.

11 Ibid., 295.

12 Donald P. Francis, 'A Plea for More Funding,' *Frontline*, accessed December 23, 2011, http://www.pbs.org/wgbh/pages/frontline/aids/docs/francisplea.html; Shilts, *And the Band*, 273.

13 Shilts, *And the Band*, 191.

14 Ibid., 110.

15 Philip Boffey, 'Reagan Defends Financing for AIDS,' *New York Times*, September 18, 1985, accessed December 23, 2011, http://www.nytimes.com/1985/09/18/us/reagan-defends-financing-for-aids.html.

16 Shilts, *And the Band*, 143.

17 Associated Press, 'AIDS Gets Mixed Response from Clergy,' *Ocala Star-Banner*, October 5, 1985, accessed January 4, 2012, http://news.google.com/newspapers?nid=1356&dat=19851005&id=-35RAAAAIBAJ&sjid=UAYEAAAAIBAJ&pg=2891,3418390.

18 Shilts, *And the Band*, 311.

19 Michael Hirsley, 'Aids Education Effort May Have

Backfired,' *Chicago Tribune*, November 10, 1985, accessed January 4, 2012, http://articles.chicagotribune.com/ 1985–11–10/news/8503170436_1_aids-victims-common-cup-blood-banks.

20 Abigail Trafford and Gordon Witkin, 'The Politics of AIDS – A Tale of Two States,' *U.S. News & World Report*, November 18, 1985.

21 Rock Hudson and Sara Davidson, *Rock Hudson: His Story* (New York: William Morrow, 1986), 158, accessed March 2, 2012, http://www.amazon.com/dp/0688064728/ ref=rdr_ext_tmb.

22 William F. Buckley, 'Crucial Steps in Combating the Aids Epidemic; Identify All the Carriers,' *New York Times*, March 18, 1986, accessed December 23, 2011, http:// www.nytimes.com/books/00/07/16/specials/ buckley-aids. html.

23 Shilts, *And the Band*, 587.

24 Ronald Reagan, 'President Reagan's amfAR Speech,' *Frontline*, accessed December 23, 2011, http://www.pbs. org/wgbh/pages/frontline/aids/docs/amfar.html.

CHAPTER 5: A CRISIS OF CARING

1 Black AIDS Institute, *Deciding Moment: The State of AIDS in Black America 2011*, accessed December 7, 2011, http://dl.dropbox.com/u/20533079/2011stateofaid sfullreport.pdf.

2 Jose A. Vargas, 'An Overwhelmed D.C. Agency Loses Count of AIDS Cases,' *Washington Post*, December 30, 2006, accessed December 7, 2011, http://www.

washingtonpost.com/wp-dyn/content/ article/2006/12/29/ AR2006122901543.html.

3 Jose A. Vargas and Darryl Fears, 'At Least 3 Percent of D.C. Residents Have HIV or AIDS, City Study Finds; Rate up 22 Percent from 2006,' *Washington Post*, March 15, 2009, accessed December 8, 2011, http://www. washingtonpost.com/wp-dyn/content/article/2009/03/14/ AR2009031402176.html.

4 Debbie Cenziper, 'Staggering Need, Striking Neglect,' *Washington Post*, October 19, 2009, accessed December 8, 2011, http://www.washingtonpost.com/wp-dyn/content/ article/2009/10/17/AR2009101701984.html.

5 Ibid.

6 Centers for Disease Control and Prevention, 'HIV and AIDS Among Gay and Bisexual Men,' accessed March 22, 2012, http://www.cdc.gov/nchhstp/newsroom/docs/ fastfacts-msm-final508comp.pdf.

7 Anne C. Spaulding, Ryan M. Seals, Matthew J. Page, Amanda K. Brzozowski, and William Rhodes, 'HIV/ AIDS Among Inmates of and Releasees from U.S. Correctional Facilities, 2006: Declining Share of Epidemic but Persistent Public Health Opportunity,' *PLoS One* (2009), accessed February 14, 2012, http:// www.plosone. org/article/info:doi/10.1371/journal.pone.0007558.

8 'Remarks by Elizabeth Glaser: July 14 Madison Square Garden, New York City,' *Washington Post*, August 25, 1992.

CHAPTER 6: CONFRONTING REALITY

1 Rachel Jewkes, Yandisa Sikweyiya, Robert Morrell, and Kristin Dunkle, 'Understanding Men's Health and Use of Violence: Interface of Rape and HIV in South Africa,' South African Medical Research Council, accessed February 12, 2012, http://www.mrc.ac.za/gender/violence_hiv.pdf.

2 Ibid.

3 Peacewomen, 'South Africa: Rape Contributes to HIV/AIDS Spread Among SADC Women and Girls,' accessed February 12, 2012, http://www.peacewomen.org/news_article.php?id=1538&type=news.

4 Médecins Sans Frontières, 'Shattered Lives: Immediate Medical Care Vital for Sexual Violence Victims,' accessed February 12, 2012, http://www.doctorswithoutborders.org/publications/article_print.cfm?id=3464.

5 David Smith, 'Quarter of Men in South Africa Admit Rape, Survey Finds,' *The Guardian*, June 17, 2009, accessed February 12, 2012, http://www.guardian.co.uk/world/2009/jun/17/south-africa-rape-survey.

6 Erving Goffman, *Stigma: Notes on the Management of Spoiled Identity* (New York: Simon & Schuster, 1963).

7 G. M. Herek, 'Illness, Stigma, and AIDS,' in *Psychological Aspects of Serious Illness* (Washington, DC: American Psychological Association, 1990), 103–50, also available online as a preprint of chapter, accessed April 24, 2012, http://psychology.ucdavis.edu/rainbow/html/AIDS_stigma_1990_pre.pdf.

8 Ibid.

9 Ibid.

10 Eddie Bruce-Jones and Lucas P. Itaborahy, 'State-Sponsored Homophobia: A World Survey of Laws Criminalising Same-Sex Sexual Acts Between Consenting Adults,' International Lesbian and Gay Association, accessed February 12, 2012, http://old.ilga.org/Statehomophobia/ILGA_State_Sponsored_Homophobia_2011.pdf.

11 International Gay and Lesbian Human Rights Commission, 'Uganda: Persecution of Lesbians and Gay Men Intensifies,' accessed February 12, 2012, http://www.iglhrc.org/cgi-bin/iowa/article/pressroom/pressrelease/517.html.

12 Human Rights Watch, 'Epidemic of Abuse: Police Harassment of HIV/AIDS Outreach Workers in India,' accessed February 12, 2012, http://www.unhcr.org/refworld/docid/3d4fc51f4.html.

13 amfAR, 'MSM and HIV/AIDS Risk in Asia: What Is Fueling the Epidemic Among MSM and How Can It Be Stopped?' accessed February 12, 2012, http://www.amfar.org/uploadedFiles/In_the_Community/Publications/MSM%20and%20HIV%20AIDS%20Risk%20in%20Asia.pdf.

14 Centers for Disease Control and Prevention, 'HIV and AIDS Among Gay and Bisexual Men,' accessed February 12, 2012, http://www.cdc.gov/nchhstp/newsroom/docs/fastfacts-msm-final508comp.pdf.

15 Steffanie A. Strathdee and David Vlahov, 'The Effectiveness of Needle Exchange Programs: A Review of the Science and Policy,' *AIDScience* 1, no. 16 (2001),

accessed February 13, 2012, http://aidscience.org/Articles/aidscience013.asp.

16 AIDS Action, 'Syringe Exchange and HIV/AIDS,' accessed March 2, 2012, http://www.aidsaction.org/attachments/518_Syringe%20Exchange.pdf.

17 'HIV Is Not a Crime, 2011 Film by Sean Strub, Edit by Leo Herrera/HomoChic,' YouTube video, 8:12, posted by 'SeanStrub,' November 30, 2011, accessed April 24, 2012, http://www.youtube.com/watch?v=iB-6blJjbjc.

18 Madison Park, 'As HIV Epidemic Grows, Florida City Grapples with Fear and Denial,' CNN, November 29, 2011, accessed February 13, 2012, http://www.cnn.com/2011/11/29/health/jacksonville-hiv-florida/index.html.

CHAPTER 7: THE HEART OF THE MATTER

1 Evgeny Lebedev, 'On the Streets with Ukraine's Lost Generation,' The Independent, December 1, 2011, accessed December 17, 2011, http://www.independent.co.uk/life-style/health-and-families/features/elton-john-on-the-streets-with-ukraines-lost-generation-6270102.html.

2 Paul Smith, 'Welcome to the Occupation,' accessed December 22, 2011, http://www.welcometotheoccupa-tion.com/2010/01/hr-carnival-to-aid-haiti-serovie.html.

3 IGLHRC/SEROvie, 'The Impact of the Earthquake and Relief and Recovery Programs on Haitian LGBT People,' accessed December 21, 2011, http://www.iglhrc.org/cgi-bin/iowa/article/publications/reportsandpublications/1369.html.

4 Ibid.

5   Ibid.

CHAPTER 8: A GREAT POWER

1   Bill Frist, *A Heart to Serve: The Passion to Bring Health, Hope, and Healing* (New York: Center Street, 2009), accessed February 13, 2012, http://books.google.com/books?id=VRg1v0jSoWUC&1pg=PT182&vq=aids&pg=PT3#v=onepage&q=1981&f=false.

2   Heather Timmons and Nikhila Gill, 'India's Health Minister Calls Homosexuality "Unnatural,"' *New York Times*, July 5, 2011, accessed February 13, 2012, http://www.nytimes.com/2011/07/06/world/asia/06india.html.

3   Sarah Boseley, 'Mbeki Aids Denial "Caused 300,000 Deaths,"' *The Guardian*, November 26, 2008, accessed February 13, 2012, http://www.guardian.co.uk/world/2008/nov/26/aids-south-africa.

4   Pride Chigwedere, George R. Seage, Sofia Gruskin, Tun-Hou Lee, and M. Essex, 'Estimating the Lost Benefits of Antiretroviral Drug Use in South Africa,' *JAIDS Journal of Acquired Immune Deficiency Syndromes* 49, no. 4 (2008): 410–15, accessed February 13, 2012, http://journals.lww.com/jaids/Fulltext/2008/12010/Estimating_the_Lost_Benefits_of_Antiretroviral.10.aspx.

5   'SA's Zuma "Showered to Avoid HIV,"' BBC News, April 5, 2006, accessed February 13, 2012, http://news.bbc.co.uk/2/hi/africa/4879822.stm.

6   Bruce Japsen, 'Budget Squeeze Could Make HIV Treatment Costlier, Rarer,' *Chicago Tribune*, February 9,

2011, accessed March 23, 2012, http://articles.chicago tribune.com/2011-02-09/business/ct-biz-0209-aids-treatment-delays-20110209_1_hiv-drugs-aids-patients-aids-drug-assistance-program.

CHAPTER 9: A GREAT RESPONSIBILITY

1 Walt Bogdanich and Eric Koli, '2 Paths of Bayer Drug in '80s: Riskier One Steered Overseas,' *New York Times*, May 22, 2003, accessed February 14, 2012, http://www. nytimes.com/2003/05/22/business/2-paths-of-bayer-drug-in-80-s-riskier-one-steered-overseas .html?pagewanted=all&src=pm.

2 Jim Edwards, 'Bayer Admits It Paid "Millions" in HIV Infection Cases – Just Not in English,' CBS News, January 28, 2011, accessed March 23, 2012, http://www .cbsnews.com/8301–505123–162–42847237/bayer-admits-it-paid-millions-in-hiv-infection-cases----just-not-in-english/.

3 Jonathan Rauch, '"This Is Not Charity,"' *The Atlantic*, October 2007, accessed February 14, 2012, http://www .theatlantic.com/magazine/archive/2007/10/-ldquo-this-is-not-charity-rdquo/6197/.

4 Ibid.

5 Celia W. Dugger, 'Clinton Foundation Announces a Bargain on Generic AIDS Drugs,' *New York Times*, May 9, 2007, accessed February 14, 2012, http://www.nytimes. com/2007/05/09/world/09aidsdrugs.html.

6 'Pope Benedict on the Use of Condoms: Book Excerpt,' BBC News, November 20, 2010, accessed February 14,

2012, http://www.bbc.co.uk/news/world-europe-11804798.

7   Ibid.

8   Vatican, 'Encyclical Letter Humanae Vitae,' accessed February 14, 2012, http://www.vatican.va/holy_father/paul_vi/encyclicals/documents/hf_p-vi_enc_25071968humanae-vitae_en.html.

9   Jonathan Clayton, 'Condom Ban by John Paul Only Escalated Crisis,' *The Australian*, March 19, 2009.

10   'Vatican: Condoms Don't Stop Aids,' *The Guardian*, October 9, 2003, accessed February 14, 2012, http://www.guardian.co.uk/world/2003/oct/09/aids.

11   Riazat Butt, 'Pope Claims Condoms Could Make African Aids Crisis Worse,' *The Guardian*, March 17, 2009, accessed February 14, 2012, http://www.guardian.co.uk/world/2009/mar/17/pope-africa-condoms-aids.

12   Nicholas D. Kristof, 'The Pope and AIDS,' *New York Times*, May 8, 2005, accessed February 14, 2012, http://www.nytimes.com/2005/05/08/opinion/08kristof.html.

13   Ibid.

CHAPTER 10: ENDING AIDS FOREVER

1   Joint United Nations Programme on HIV/AIDS, 'A New Investment Framework for the Global HIV Response,' accessed March 15, 2012, http://www.unaids.org/en/media/unaids/contentassets/documents/unaidspublication/2011/JC2244_InvestmentFramework_en.pdf.

2   UNAIDS, 'World AIDS Day Report 2011,' accessed March 23, 2012, http://www.unaids.org/en/media/unaids/

contentassets/documents/unaidspublication/2011/
JC2216_WorldAIDSday_report_2011_en.pdf.

3   Jennifer Kates, Adam Wexler, Eric Lief, Carlos Avila, and
Benjamin Gobet, 'Financing the Response to AIDS in
Low- and Middle-Income Countries: International
Assistance from Donor Governments in 2010,' UNAIDS
and Kaiser Family Foundation, accessed April 18, 2012,
http://www.kff.org/hivaids/upload/7347–07.pdf.

About the Author

The monumental career of international singer-song-writer and performer Sir Elton John has spanned more than five decades. He is one of the top-selling solo artists of all time, with thirty-five Gold and twenty-five Platinum albums and twenty-nine consecutive Top 40 hits, and he has sold more than 250 million records worldwide. Elton holds the record for the biggest-selling single of all time, 'Candle in the Wind,' which sold 37 million copies. The National Academy of Recording Arts and Sciences has awarded Elton five Grammys and the Grammy Legend Award, and honoured him with the MusiCares Person of the Year Award. Elton was inducted into the Rock and Roll Hall of Fame in 1994. Additionally, he was the first artist honoured by the Billboard Touring Conference with its Legend of Live Award, which recognises those in the concert business who have made a significant and lasting impact on the industry. And in September 2013, Elton was honoured as the first recipient of the prestigious BRITs Icon Award. He continues to tour all over the world. Elton was honoured with a commemorative banner during his sixtieth performance at Madison Square Garden for the 'Most Performances by a Single Artist' at the legendary venue. His induction into Madison Square Garden's Music Hall of Fame coincided with his sixtieth birthday. In September 2011 Elton began a three-year residency at the Colosseum at Caesars Palace in Las Vegas with an all-new show, *The Million Dollar Piano*.

His album with Leon Russell, *The Union*, produced by T-Bone Burnett, was released in October 2010 to rave reviews. The first single was nominated for a Grammy for Best Pop Collaboration with Vocals. In April 2011 the Tribeca Film Festival opened with the world premiere of Cameron Crowe's documentary *The Union*, which features the writing and recording of the Elton John and Leon Russell album. Elton's collaboration with T Bone Burnett continued in September 2013 when he released *The Diving Board*, his first studio album in seven years, to rave reviews. The album features 12 new songs written by Elton and his longtime lyricist Bernie Taupin.

The smash-hit stage production of *Billy Elliot*, for which Elton composed the music, originally opened in London and garnered him a top-five hit in the UK with the song 'Electricity.' *Billy Elliot* was nominated for a record nine Olivier Awards, winning Best Musical, among others. It opened on Broadway on November 13, 2008, to critical acclaim. It was nominated for a record-tying fifteen Tony Awards and won ten, including Best Musical. In March 2011 *Billy Elliot* opened in Toronto to rave reviews.

Elton received an Academy Award for *The Lion King* and Tony Awards for both *The Lion King* and *Aida*. He served as the executive producer for the hugely successful animated feature *Gnomeo & Juliet*, which opened in February 2011.

In 1992, Elton established the Elton John AIDS Foundation (EJAF), which today is one of the leading non-profit HIV/AIDS organisations. EJAF has raised $275 million to date to support hundreds of HIV/AIDS prevention and service programmes around the globe. In 1998, the queen of England knighted him Sir Elton John, CBE. In 2004, he received Kennedy Center Honors for his lifetime contributions to American culture and excellence through the performing arts. In 2013, in recognition of his philanthropic and humanitarian efforts through EJAF, Elton received the Harvard School of Public Health AIDS Initiative Leadership Award and the Rockefeller Foundation's Lifetime Achievement Award.

Index